Resistance Bands Exercises

FOR SENIORS OVER 70

Quick and Simple Low-Impact Workouts to Build Strength, Balance and Mobility

DR. DANIEL BYARS

DISCLAIMER

The information contained in this book is intended for educational and informational purposes only. It is not a substitute for professional medical advice, diagnosis, or treatment. Always seek the advice of your physician or other qualified health provider with any questions you may have regarding a medical condition or exercise program.

The author is not responsible for any injuries or damages that may arise from the use of the information provided in this book. Readers are encouraged to consult with their healthcare provider before beginning any new exercise regimen, especially if they have pre-existing health conditions or concerns.

TABLE OF CONTENTS

Disclaimer... 2

About The Author 6

What Readers Are Saying 8

Introduction 10

Chapter 1: Understanding The Advantages Of Resistance Bands For Seniors 16

An Overview Of Resistance Band Exercise And Why It Is Beneficial For Seniors 16

How Resistance Bands Enhance Balance, Flexibility, And Mobility 23

Practical Applications Of Resistance Bands... 28

Promoting Joint Health And Reducing The Risk Of Injury....................... 30

Chapter 2: Getting Started (Choosing The Right Resistance Bands) 36

Choosing The Right Resistance Band For Your Fitness Level 36

Where To Buy Resistance Bands... 43

Safety Tips For Using Resistance Bands... 50

Creating A Comfortable Workout Space... 57

Chapter 3: Preparing Your Body For Exercise............................ **64**

The Value Of Warm-Up Routines For Seniors.............................. *64*

Simple Stretching And Mobility Exercises With Resistance Bands........... *71*

How To Avoid Muscle Strain And Injury.................................... *79*

Chapter 4: Resistance Band Exercises For Beginners.................... **86**

Chapter 5: Resistance Band Exercises For Intermediates **92**

Chapter 6: Seated Resistance Band Exercises **98**

Chapter 7: Resistance Band Exercises For Advanced Level **104**

Chapter 8: Rounding Off With Full-Body Exercises......................**110**

Chapter 9: Staying Motivated And Overcoming Challenges **116**

Tips For Maintaining Consistency With Your Exercise Routine.............. *116*

Working Around Common Obstacles: Pain, Fatigue, And A Lack Of Time
.... *122*

Real-Life Testimonies And Success Stories To Inspire *127*

Chapter 10: Cool Down And Recovery..................................**134**

The Importance Of Cooling Down After Workouts................................. *134*

Breathing Techniques For Post-Workout Recovery *139*

Managing Soreness And Preventing Overexertion In Seniors.................. *144*

Conclusion **150**

ABOUT THE AUTHOR

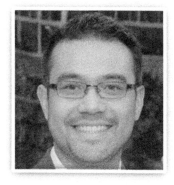 *Dr. Daniel Byars* is a dedicated **health and wellness practitioner** with over a decade of experience in fitness and rehabilitation of all ages. He holds a Doctorate in Physical Therapy and has spent his career specializing in helping individuals of all ages to maintain their strength, mobility, and independence through safe and effective exercise programs.

Passionate about empowering older adults, Dr. Byars has worked in various settings, including hospitals, rehabilitation centers, and community programs. He understands the unique challenges seniors face regarding physical activity and is committed to providing practical solutions that enhance quality of life. His approach combines evidence-based practices with a deep understanding of the aging process, making him a trusted resource for seniors and their families.

Dr. Byars is also a sought-after speaker and educator, frequently leading workshops and seminars on the benefits of exercise for older adults. He believes that fitness is a lifelong journey and strives to inspire his clients and readers to embrace movement, no matter their age or ability.

When he's not working, Dr. Byars enjoys hiking, reading, and spending quality time with his family. He lives in a small town with his wife and two active children, who keep him motivated to stay fit and engaged.

What Readers Are Saying

Robert M. from New York

I have struggled with my mobility for years, and I never thought I could get back to exercising. After reading this book, I was inspired by Evelyn's story and felt motivated to try resistance bands. The gentle approach is perfect for my needs, and I have already noticed improvements in my strength and energy levels.

Helen T. from Illinois

What a wonderful resource for seniors! The exercises are simple yet effective, and I love the focus on safety. I have shared this book with my friends and even started a little exercise group together, all thanks to your guidance.

George P. from Washington

This book changed my life! I had given up on staying active after my surgery, but the practical tips and encouragement I found on these pages inspired me to give resistance bands a try. I feel stronger and more balanced than I have in years. Thank you for this invaluable resource.

INTRODUCTION

Our freedom and vigor may be hampered by the increased difficulties we frequently encounter as we age. As we manage these changes, maintaining strength, balance, and mobility is critical not only for physical health but also for general well-being. Regardless of where you are beginning from, this masterpiece is meant to give you the confidence to take charge of your fitness path.

Resistance bands are simple, adaptable, and effective equipment that can substantially improve your strength training regimen. Unlike traditional weights, resistance bands provide a wide range of motion and can be readily modified to meet individual demands, making them ideal for seniors. This book will teach you how to use resistance bands to build strength, improve flexibility, and improve balance—all of which are necessary for good aging.

*To demonstrate the significant impact of resistance band training, consider the remarkable story of **Evelyn Carter,** a lively lady in her 70s. Evelyn struggled with the physical changes that frequently accompany aging after retiring from a fulfilling profession. Weight gain, diminished mobility, and increasing frustration began to eclipse her golden years. Like* *many others, she was overwhelmed by the idea of restoring her health.*

Evelyn's turning point occurred when she was introduced to resistance band exercises at her local community center. Initially hesitant, she soon realized that these bands could deliver an efficient, low-impact workout that would integrate perfectly into her routine. Resistance bands' adaptability enabled her to undertake a range of exercises that targeted different muscle areas while remaining easy on her joints. She began with simple moves and worked her way up to more difficult routines, enjoying the steady gains in her strength and balance.

Evelyn's physical fitness improved, and she saw improvements that went beyond the physical. She gained confidence as she felt more in control of her body and health. She was able to participate in things she had previously enjoyed but had avoided owing to physical restrictions, such as gardening and playing with her grandkids. The beneficial impacts spread throughout her life, improving her emotional well-being and inspiring her to share her experiences with others.

Evelyn's metamorphosis is a striking demonstration of the benefits of resistance band training. Her experience serves as a reminder that it's never too late to start living a healthier, more vibrant life. This book seeks to provide you with the same tools and direction that Evelyn used to restore her strength, balance, and mobility.

In this book, you will learn about the different types of resistance bands and how to choose the best one for your fitness level. Each chapter is designed to provide clear directions for a range of exercises, beginning with warm-ups and advancing to beginner, intermediate, and advanced routines. This organized technique helps you to steadily improve your skills while avoiding the risks of injury or dissatisfaction.

One of the primary advantages of resistance bands is their low-impact nature. Seniors can now engage in strength training without concern about injuring their muscles or joints. Resistance bands operate by supplying resistance in both directions, thereby improving muscular coordination and balance. This is especially crucial for the elderly because falls and injuries can have a substantial impact on their quality of life.

Throughout this book, you will also learn how to tailor your fitness regimen to your specific needs. Each individual's experience is unique, and I understand that one size does not fit all. You'll learn how to combine strength, flexibility, and balance exercises in a method that feels comfortable for you.

As you procced through the chapters, you will come across real-life testimonies from seniors who have adopted resistance band training. These stories demonstrate not just physical changes, but also mental and social benefits from regular exercise. Resistance band training has a significant impact on everything from regaining the capacity to engage in family activities to feeling empowered to undertake new experiences.

As you embark on this path, realize that transformation takes time. Celebrate minor accomplishments, and don't be afraid to adapt exercises as needed. Always listen to your body and put safety first. The goal is development, not perfection, and each step toward greater strength, balance, and mobility is worth celebrating.

This book is more than just exercises; it is about cultivating an attitude of resilience and empowerment. It is about accepting the opportunities that come with living an active lifestyle as we age. With each chapter, I want you to imagine a future in which you can walk confidently, enjoy your everyday activities, and possibly even inspire others to take control of their health.

This book is your path to regaining your strength and mobility. It contains useful information, expert advice, and a variety of exercises tailored just for you. As you turn the pages and interact with the exercises, consider it a journey toward vitality similar to Evelyn Carter's.

Whether you are an experienced fitness enthusiast or just starting, this book will provide you with the tools you need to succeed. Remember, every hour you spend on your health is an investment in your future. Let's start our adventure together, one resistance band exercise at a time. Your next chapter of strength, balance, and mobility awaits.

CHAPTER 1: UNDERSTANDING THE ADVANTAGES OF RESISTANCE BANDS FOR SENIORS

An Overview Of Resistance Band Exercise And Why It Is Beneficial For Seniors

Resistance band training has become popular in recent years as a simple but extremely efficient method of exercise for people of all fitness levels, particularly seniors. This adaptable training method employs elastic bands to provide resistance during movement, thereby strengthening muscles, improving flexibility, and increasing total mobility. Resistance bands provide seniors with a practical, safe, and accessible way to maintain or enhance their physical fitness without the use of heavy equipment or intricate routines. This type of exercise has been shown to improve strength, balance, and joint health, making it excellent for people over 70 who wish to remain active, healthy, and independent.

Resistance bands are elastic bands available in a range of sizes, forms, and resistance levels. They are lightweight, portable, and affordable, making them a viable alternative to traditional weightlifting or gym activities. Bands are classified according to the amount of resistance they provide—light, medium, or heavy—and can be used to target different muscle areas depending on how they are positioned or attached. Some bands include handles or loops, while others are only strips of elastic cloth. Resistance bands, regardless of their construction, enable users to execute a variety of workouts that replicate the benefits of weight training while putting little strain on the joints.

Why Resistance Band Training is Beneficial for Seniors

Maintaining strength, balance, and mobility as we get older is critical to our general health and freedom. Resistance band training is an excellent option for seniors over 70 to achieve their fitness goals while avoiding the hazards associated with high-impact or severe activity. Here are a few reasons why this form of training is ideal for older folks.

1. Low-impact, joint-friendly

One of the most significant advantages of resistance band exercise for seniors is its moderate impact. Resistance band activities are gentler on the body than high-impact exercises like jogging or leaping, which can stress the joints and cause damage. This is especially crucial for seniors who have arthritis, joint discomfort, or other age-related diseases that prevent them from engaging in more strenuous physical activity. Seniors can use resistance bands to increase their strength and flexibility without worsening their existing joint difficulties.

In addition to being low-impact, resistance bands provide a controlled kind of resistance, allowing seniors to gradually increase the intensity of their workouts as their muscles strengthen. This allows you to gradually gain muscle and maintain joint health without risking overexertion or injury.

2. Improves strength without using heavy weights

Strength training is vital for seniors to preserve muscular mass, which naturally decreases as they age. Sarcopenia, or muscle mass loss, can cause a deterioration in physical function, making daily chores like carrying groceries, climbing stairs, or even rising from a chair more difficult. Resistance band workouts target major muscle areas, allowing seniors to gain and maintain strength without the need for heavy weights or gym equipment.

Resistance bands are especially useful for seniors because they may be changed depending on the individual's fitness level. Light resistance bands are ideal for beginners or those recovering from an injury, whilst larger bands can provide a more challenging workout for seniors who are ready to develop. This resistance-level flexibility allows seniors to continually push their muscles and avoid plateaus in their exercise path.

3. Improves balance and stability

Falls are a major worry for seniors, with balance and stability concerns being the main cause of injury in older persons. Resistance band exercise can assist improve balance by strengthening the muscles that support the body's core, hips, and legs—important areas for stability. Exercises that target specific muscle groups can lower the likelihood of falling and improve general coordination.

Exercises like the standing row or banded side steps, for example, target the muscles responsible for balance, assisting seniors in developing improved posture and physical control. Over time, these exercises can help seniors move with confidence, whether they are walking, climbing stairs, or doing other daily activities.

Incorporating balance-focused resistance band exercises into a regular workout regimen can improve a senior's ability to stay steady on their feet, lowering the chance of falls and injuries.

4. Improves flexibility and range of motion

Maintaining flexibility and range of motion is an important part of exercise for seniors. As we age, our muscles and joints harden, resulting in decreased mobility and difficulty completing basic actions. Resistance bands are a fantastic tool for stretching and developing flexibility because they allow seniors to go through their whole range of motion while providing just enough resistance to gently stretch muscles.

Seniors can improve their range of motion by completing flexibility exercises daily, such as seated leg lifts or seated hamstring stretches. This makes everyday actions like bending, reaching, and turning simpler and less uncomfortable. Improved flexibility also reduces muscle strain and prevents injuries, allowing elders to maintain an active lifestyle.

5. Promotes independence and functional fitness

Functional fitness workouts are those that mirror the motions used during daily activity. Maintaining functional fitness is crucial for seniors who want to keep their independence and quality of life. Resistance band workouts are intended to increase the strength and coordination required to execute daily tasks like lifting objects, standing up, and walking.

Exercises like the seated chest press and banded squats target the muscles engaged in activities like getting out of a chair, carrying groceries, and reaching for items on a high shelf. Resistance band training, which focuses on functional motions, can help seniors maintain their physical ability to accomplish daily tasks with ease, extending their independence and lowering the need for assistance.

6. Portable and convenient to use anywhere

Resistance band training is also great for seniors because it is portable and simple to use. Unlike huge training machines or free weights, resistance bands are portable and may be used in almost any place. Seniors can simply add resistance band workouts into their daily routines at home, in the park, or when traveling, without the need for a designated workout space or pricey gym fees.

Because they are so convenient, resistance bands make it easier for seniors to stick to their training routine. Regular exercise is essential for long-term health, and the simplicity of resistance bands removes many typical hurdles to keeping active, such as time constraints, a lack of equipment, or difficulties traveling to the gym.

7. Cost-effective and accessible

For many elders, pricey gym equipment or personal trainers may not be an option. Resistance bands are an affordable option that nevertheless provides considerable exercise advantages. They are reasonable and readily available, allowing seniors to invest in their health without breaking their pocketbook.

Furthermore, resistance band exercises are easy to master and require no training. Many senior citizens can do these exercises at home with the help of an instructional book, video, or fitness professional. This accessibility means that seniors of all fitness levels can begin resistance band training and receive the advantages without feeling overwhelmed or frightened.

Resistance band training is a comprehensive option for seniors seeking to improve their strength, balance, flexibility, and overall physical health. Its low-impact, joint-friendly nature makes it perfect for older folks, particularly those with pre-existing health conditions or limited mobility. Seniors who incorporate resistance band exercises into their fitness program can maintain independence, lower the chance of injury, and improve their quality of life well into their later years.

How Resistance Bands Enhance Balance, Flexibility, And Mobility

Maintaining our physical health becomes more vital as we become older, especially for seniors over 70. Resistance bands are a highly effective technique for increasing strength and promoting general fitness in this demographic. These adaptable pieces of equipment provide a low-impact way to engage in strength training while also considerably improving balance, flexibility, and mobility.

Before getting into the specific benefits of resistance bands, it's important to grasp what balance, flexibility, and mobility mean.

Balance is the capacity to maintain one's position while fixed or moving. Good balance is essential for daily tasks, as it reduces the danger of falls and improves stability.

Flexibility is the range of motion in a joint or collection of joints. Increased flexibility aids in daily chores, improves posture and lowers the likelihood of injury.

Mobility refers to the capacity to move freely and easily. This comprises functional movement patterns necessary for daily activities such as walking, bending, and climbing stairs.

Resistance bands are elastic bands that produce variable degrees of resistance when stretched. They come in a variety of shapes, sizes, and strengths, making them appropriate for persons at various fitness levels. The next sections explain how resistance bands improve balance, flexibility, and mobility.

1. Improving Balance

❖ ***Strengthening and stabilizing muscles:*** Balance is primarily dependent on the power of stabilizing muscles, which help us maintain our posture and stay upright. Resistance bands make it easier to perform activities that specifically target certain muscles. Exercises like the Banded Side Step and Standing Row, for example, need the core, hips, and legs to be activated, which improves stability.

❖ ***Dynamic balance training:*** Resistance bands can also be utilized to do dynamic balance workouts. For example, using a resistance band to perform a movement like the Single Leg Deadlift requires the body to engage stabilizing muscles in order to maintain balance. This dynamic exercise is essential for elders because it resembles real-life scenarios in which keeping balance is required, such as walking on uneven ground.

❖ ***Increased proprioception:*** Proprioception is the body's ability to detect its position and movement in space. Resistance band workouts with several planes of motion improve proprioception because they demand awareness of body positioning. Improved proprioception leads to better balance and coordination, which reduces the risk of falling.

2. Enhancing Flexibility

❖ *Gently stretching using resistance bands:* One of the most significant advantages of resistance bands is their ability to aid in stretching exercises that improve flexibility. Unlike static stretching, which can put strain on joints and muscles, resistance bands allow for controlled, mild stretches. Resistance band exercises, such as the Seated Hamstring Stretch and Standing Chest Stretch, can be used to gradually stretch muscles and increase flexibility.

❖ *Targeting specific muscle groups:* Resistance bands allow seniors to target certain muscle areas effectively. This specialized technique helps to improve flexibility in certain parts of the body, such as the hips, shoulders, and back. Exercises such as the Seated Shoulder Press and Seated Leg Lift can be performed with bands to increase flexibility in these areas and promote a wider range of motion.

❖ *Reducing muscle tension:* Regular stretching with resistance bands helps to relieve muscle stress and tightness, which are typical with aging. Seniors who incorporate resistance band workouts into their routines can maintain muscle suppleness and joint flexibility, reducing stiffness and discomfort.

3. Promoting Mobility

❖ *Functional movement patterns:* Resistance bands are ideal for developing functional movement patterns, which are required to preserve mobility in daily life. Exercises like the Chest Press and Lateral Raises mirror motions found in ordinary life, such as reaching for goods or lifting stuff. Training these movements helps elders keep their independence and carry out daily tasks more easily.

❖ *Incorporating full-body movements:* Many resistance band workouts include various muscle groups, which improves general mobility. For example, a Banded Squat strengthens the legs while simultaneously engaging the core and improving coordination. Seniors can improve their overall functional capacity by including full-body exercises in their workouts, making it simpler to shift from sitting to standing to walking.

❖ *Boosting joint health:* Resistance band exercise is low-impact, making it easier on the joints than traditional weightlifting. This feature is especially important for the elderly who may suffer from joint pain or arthritis. Resistance bands help to strengthen the muscles around joints, providing better support and stability, which improves mobility and reduces the likelihood of injury.

Practical Applications Of Resistance Bands

Seniors can use resistance bands efficiently to improve balance, flexibility, and mobility by following a systematic regimen. Here are a few practical applications:

1. *Balanced Routine:* Use exercises like Banded Side Steps and Single Leg Raises to activate stabilizing muscles. Exercises like Standing Rows require you to maintain balance while completing upper-body movements.

2. *Flexible Routine:* Use bands for gentle stretching activities like seated hamstring stretches and standing quadriceps stretches. Include resistance band practices that combine dynamic stretching to enhance flexibility across several muscle groups.

3. *Mobility Routine:* To improve mobility, use functional movement exercises like banded squats and chest presses. Include exercises that replicate daily tasks, which will help to reinforce movement patterns and enhance mobility.

Resistance bands are a helpful tool for seniors looking to improve their balance, flexibility, and mobility. Resistance bands offer a complete approach to physical health by providing focused exercises that strengthen stabilizing muscles, encourage moderate stretching, and support functional movement patterns.

Seniors who add resistance band training into their routines may find an enhanced quality of life, more independence, and a lower risk of falls and accidents. Focusing on these important areas can help seniors stay active and engaged in their everyday activities, boosting longevity and well-being.

Promoting Joint Health And Reducing The Risk Of Injury

Joint health is crucial for maintaining overall mobility and quality of life, especially as we age. Our joints allow us to perform everyday activities such as walking, climbing stairs, and even simple tasks like reaching for an object. As we age, the risk of joint-related issues increases, leading to conditions such as arthritis, joint pain, and reduced mobility. Promoting joint health and minimizing the risk of injury is essential to maintaining an active and fulfilling lifestyle.

Joints are the points where two or more bones meet, and they are critical for movement. They are made up of several components, including cartilage, ligaments, tendons, and synovial fluid. Cartilage is a smooth tissue that covers the ends of bones in a joint, allowing for smooth movement and acting as a cushion to absorb shock. Ligaments are tough, fibrous tissues that connect bones, while tendons attach muscles to bones. Synovial fluid is a viscous liquid that lubricates joints, reducing friction and aiding in smooth movement.

As we age, the cartilage in our joints can wear down, leading to pain, stiffness, and inflammation. Conditions such as osteoarthritis, rheumatoid arthritis, and bursitis can develop, significantly affecting mobility and overall quality of life.

Therefore, understanding how to promote joint health and reduce the risk of injury is vital.

Key Strategies for Promoting Joint Health

1. Regular Exercise

Regular physical activity is one of the most effective ways to maintain joint health. Engaging in low-impact exercises, such as walking, swimming, and cycling, can help strengthen the muscles around the joints, improve flexibility, and enhance overall joint function. Resistance training, particularly with tools like resistance bands, can provide safe strength-building workouts that protect joints while promoting muscle strength.

Stretching exercises can also improve flexibility and range of motion in the joints. Incorporating activities like yoga or tai chi can enhance balance and stability, reducing the risk of falls and injuries.

2. Maintaining a Healthy Weight

Excess weight places additional stress on weight-bearing joints, particularly the knees, hips, and spine. Maintaining a healthy weight through a balanced diet and regular exercise can significantly reduce the risk of joint pain and injury. Even a modest weight loss of 5-10% can alleviate pressure on the joints and improve overall joint health.

3. Balanced Nutrition

A nutritious diet plays a critical role in joint health. Consuming foods rich in omega-3 fatty acids, such as fish, flaxseeds, and walnuts, can help reduce inflammation in the joints. Antioxidant-rich foods, such as fruits and vegetables, can combat oxidative stress and promote joint health. Vitamins and minerals like vitamin D and calcium are vital for maintaining strong bones and preventing osteoporosis, a condition that can lead to joint problems.

Staying hydrated is equally important, as adequate hydration helps maintain synovial fluid levels in the joints. A well-hydrated body is better equipped to cushion and lubricate joints, reducing friction and wear.

4. Proper Body Mechanics

Learning how to use proper body mechanics during daily activities can significantly reduce the risk of injury. When lifting objects, it is essential to bend at the knees rather than the waist and to keep the object close to the body. Using ergonomic tools and aids can also help maintain proper posture and reduce strain on the joints during repetitive tasks.

5. Incorporating Rest and Recovery

While regular exercise is essential for joint health, rest and recovery are equally important. Overuse of joints can lead to injuries such as tendonitis or bursitis. Allowing time for recovery and incorporating rest days into an exercise routine can prevent excessive strain on the joints. Listening to your body is key; if an activity causes pain, it's important to modify or stop the movement.

6. Utilizing Joint Support Tools

In some cases, using supportive devices such as braces or splints can help stabilize and protect joints, especially if there is a history of injury or discomfort. These tools can provide added support during physical activity, helping to prevent injury and promoting safe movement.

Reducing the Risk of Injury

1. *Warm-Up and Cool-Down:* Always start a workout with a warm-up to prepare your muscles and joints for exercise. Warming up increases blood flow and improves flexibility, reducing the risk of injury. After exercising, cooling down with gentle stretches helps prevent stiffness and promotes recovery.

2. *Recognizing and Addressing Pain:* Pain is the body's way of signaling that something is wrong. Ignoring pain can lead to further injury. It's important to recognize the difference between muscle soreness and joint pain. If you experience persistent joint pain, seek medical advice to address the underlying cause.

3. *Modifying Activities:* When it comes aging, it's essential to modify activities to match our current fitness levels and joint health. This may involve adjusting the intensity of workouts, choosing low-impact alternatives, or utilizing supportive equipment.

4. *Staying Informed:* Educating oneself about joint health, injury prevention, and proper exercise techniques can empower individuals to take proactive steps in maintaining their well-being. Attending workshops, consulting fitness professionals, or reading reputable sources on joint health can provide valuable insights.

Promoting joint health and reducing the risk of injury are essential components of a healthy, active lifestyle, especially for seniors. By incorporating regular exercise, maintaining a healthy weight, eating a balanced diet, using proper body mechanics, and allowing for rest and recovery, individuals can support their joints and enhance their overall quality of life.

Awareness of body signals, along with a commitment to joint health, can empower seniors to remain active, independent, and injury-free. Investing time and effort into joint care today can lead to a healthier tomorrow, allowing individuals to continue enjoying the activities they love.

CHAPTER 2: GETTING STARTED (CHOOSING THE RIGHT RESISTANCE BANDS)

Choosing The Right Resistance Band For Your Fitness Level

To gain the maximum benefits of resistance band exercises, choose the appropriate band for your fitness level. Using the proper resistance band ensures that you are effectively exercising your muscles while avoiding damage.

Resistance bands exist in a variety of styles, each with a different level of resistance. The resistance level is often represented by the color of the band, which varies by manufacturer. While the color-coding method isn't consistent across all brands, here's a rough breakdown of resistance band levels:

1. *Light Resistance Bands:* These bands provide the least resistance and are commonly used by novices or those recovering from an injury. They are also appropriate for the elderly with reduced mobility or those just beginning a workout regimen.

2. *Medium Resistance Bands:* These offer moderate resistance and are perfect for people with a basic level of fitness who want to push themselves a little further. Medium bands promote muscle tone and strength without being too difficult.

3. *Heavy Resistance Bands:* These are intended for more advanced users who have established a firm foundation of strength and wish to improve their resistance training. Seniors who have been exercising regularly and are comfortable with lesser resistance bands can go to heavier ones for increased muscle engagement.

4. *Extra Heavy Resistance Bands:* These are rarely advised for seniors unless they have extensive fitness experience. Athletes and others seeking rigorous strength training frequently utilize very heavy bands. For the majority of seniors, lighter or medium resistance bands will provide an adequate challenge without causing strain or injury.

5. *Loop Bands:* These bands make a continuous loop and are commonly used for lower-body workouts like glute work and leg strengthening. Loop bands are ideal for specific exercises that improve balance and stability.

6. *Therapy Bands:* These bands are often thinner and offer lower amounts of resistance. They are frequently utilized in

physical therapy settings, making them perfect for seniors recovering from injury or surgery. Therapy bands are soft on joints and muscles, making them an appropriate choice for beginners or individuals with special physical restrictions.

Factors to Consider When Choosing a Resistance Band

Choosing the right resistance band is more than just picking a color; it's also important to evaluate your current fitness level, goals, and comfort with different workouts. The following are the essential variables to consider while selecting a resistance band.

1. Assess your fitness level

The resistance band that is best for you depends on your current strength, flexibility, and workout experience. If you're just getting started, a mild resistance band is the most secure option. This allows you to complete the exercises correctly while reducing the chance of damage.

Medium resistance bands may be an appropriate level of challenge for seniors who have been exercising frequently and are confident in their abilities. They generate more tension than light bands, allowing you to increase strength and endurance without overworking your muscles.

If you've been using resistance bands for a while and are familiar with the exercises, you might want to try heavier resistance bands to increase the intensity of your workouts.

2. Know your goals

The resistance band you choose should be in line with your fitness goals. For example, if your primary goal is to enhance mobility and flexibility, lighter bands are frequently preferable because they allow for a wider range of motion while putting less strain on your joints.

If you want to gain strength, especially in the upper or lower body, medium to heavy bands may be a better option. They provide the essential tension for muscular development while still allowing for safe, low-impact exercises.

Loop bands are a wonderful option for seniors who want to improve their balance and stability. They give focused resistance to the lower body, which helps to build muscles that aid with balance and prevent falls.

3. Consider the types of exercises

The level of resistance required varies depending on the workout. For example, exercises aimed at smaller muscular areas, such as the arms and shoulders, may necessitate the use of thinner resistance bands. This allows for controlled movement and good technique without overstretching the smaller muscles.

Medium or heavy resistance bands may be more suited to exercises that target greater muscle groups, such as the legs and back. These muscles can withstand more resistance, therefore utilizing a heavier band will allow you to get better exercise for strength and endurance.

Several bands may be required for full-body training. You may use a lighter band for warm-ups and stretching, then a medium or heavy band for the primary strength-building activities.

4. Listen to your body

The easiest way to know if a resistance band is right for you is to pay attention to how your body feels during the workouts. If the band is too tight or you're having trouble doing the exercises correctly, it may be too advanced for your fitness level. In this instance, it is preferable to use a lighter band to avoid harm.

Conversely, if the workouts feel too easy and there is little resistance, it may be time to move on to a heavier band. The trick is to pick a band that provides enough resistance to push your muscles while avoiding overexertion or bad form.

5. Test the resistance

It is generally a good idea to test a band's resistance level before using it for workouts. Begin with a few simple movements, such as bicep curls or chest pulls, to test how the band feels. You should be able to finish the exercise with regulated and consistent tension throughout the range of motion.

If you feel resistance throughout the exercise and can maintain proper posture and technique, you've most likely chosen the correct band. If the band seems too loose or too tight, try adjusting the resistance level.

6. Start slowly and progress gradually

For seniors, particularly those who are new to exercise, it is critical to begin slowly and gradually increase the intensity. Begin with a light resistance band and work on perfecting the movements with the appropriate technique. As your strength grows, you can graduate to a medium band, and potentially a heavy band if you're ready for a more difficult challenge.

The idea is to build gradually. Jumping to a heavier resistance band too quickly can cause strain or injury, especially for older persons with joint or muscular issues. Resistance band training requires patience and persistence to be effective over time.

By choosing the right resistance band for your fitness level, you may safely and effectively improve your strength, balance, and mobility. This guarantees that your workouts are both difficult and fun, allowing you to remain active and independent well into your senior years.

Where To Buy Resistance Bands

When it comes to implementing resistance bands into a senior exercise program, one of the most crucial initial stages is determining where to buy high-quality bands that fulfill your requirements. Fortunately, resistance bands are widely accessible from a variety of merchants, both online and in-store. However, not all resistance bands are created equal, and it is critical to ensure that you are purchasing gear that is safe, durable, and appropriate for your activity.

1. Online retailers

One of the most convenient ways to get resistance bands is via online stores. Shopping online gives you access to a large selection of products, making it easy to compare different brands, materials, and resistance levels. Here are some of the most popular web platforms for finding resistance bands:

Amazon

Amazon is among the most extensive internet marketplaces. It provides a wide selection of resistance bands from numerous manufacturers, including well-known fitness brands and low-cost ones. Shopping on Amazon allows you to read customer reviews, compare costs, and filter by brand, material, and resistance level. Additionally, Amazon frequently has speedy shipping choices, which is beneficial for seniors who may want to have the bands sent directly to their homes.

When shopping from Amazon, it is critical to read the product descriptions thoroughly. Pay attention to the bands' thickness, length, and resistance levels to ensure they satisfy your fitness requirements. Customer reviews can also provide information about the bands' long-term durability and performance.

Fitness Equipment Websites

Many fitness equipment manufacturers and companies sell resistance bands through their dedicated websites. Companies such as TRX, Rogue Fitness, and Theraband sell high-quality resistance bands that are specifically developed for strength training, rehabilitation, and flexibility activities. These sites frequently provide more thorough information about product specs and applications than general online marketplaces.

Buying directly from a recognized fitness brand might provide you with peace of mind because you know you're getting a long-lasting, safe product. Some fitness businesses also provide instructional videos or training manuals to help you make the most of your purchase.

eBay

If you want to buy resistance bands at a lower cost, eBay is an excellent alternative. Many vendors on eBay sell both new and old exercise equipment, frequently at lower prices than retail establishments. However, while buying on eBay, be sure the seller has a reputable reputation and the goods are in new or like-new condition. Resistance bands can lose elasticity over time, lowering their effectiveness and even increasing the risk of breaking.

Specialty Fitness Retailers

Gyms, rehabilitation facilities, and fitness lovers rely on websites such as Perform Better and Power Systems to source professional-grade exercise equipment. These stores frequently stock therapeutic resistance bands, which are perfect for seniors who want low-impact strength training or recuperation exercises. While these solutions may be more expensive, superior quality ensures longer life and performance.

2. Physical establishments

Seniors who want to see and feel the product before purchasing can benefit from visiting a physical store. Many local stores sell resistance bands, and interacting with salespeople will help you ensure that you're getting the proper ones for your needs.

Sports Goods Stores

Dick's Sporting Goods, Academy Sports, and Big 5 all sell resistance bands in a range of lengths and difficulty levels. These stores usually have departments dedicated to exercise equipment, so you can compare the bands in person. In some circumstances, sales colleagues can advise you on the appropriate bands for your specific needs and fitness level.

Buying resistance bands from a sporting goods store is helpful for people who do not want to wait for shipping. You can also immediately examine the material quality to ensure that the bands are long-lasting and comfortable to wear.

Big Box retailers

Resistance bands are available at large chain retailers such as Walmart, Target, and Costco, particularly in the health and wellness or sporting goods areas. While the selection may be limited compared to what you'll find online or in specialty stores, these retailers usually provide low-cost choices that are ideal for beginners or those searching for a quick and easy answer.

Some of these stores also sell multi-packs of resistance bands, which may comprise bands with varied resistance levels. This allows you to gradually ramp up the difficulty of your workouts as you gain strength and confidence.

Pharmacy and Health Supply Stores

Local pharmacies like CVS and Walgreens, as well as specialty health supply stores, frequently stock therapeutic resistance bands. These bands are often used for rehabilitative activities and may have less resistance than what you would find at a sporting goods store. This can be an excellent alternative for seniors who are recuperating from an injury or require low-intensity bands.

In some situations, your healthcare physician may recommend a specific type or brand of resistance band that can be purchased at these locations. The bands supplied in pharmacies frequently include instructions for specific exercises, which can be useful for seniors who are new to resistance training.

3. Physical therapy clinics and gymnasiums

Seniors who already work with a physical therapist or trainer can frequently recommend or purchase high-quality resistance bands directly. Many physical therapy clinics and gyms provide resistance bands for therapeutic and exercise use, and they may sell them to their clientele.

This is a good alternative for individuals who are concerned about purchasing the wrong sort of band, as a therapist or trainer may assist you in selecting the appropriate product based on your fitness level and health requirements. In rare situations, your physical therapist may even include resistance bands as part of your recovery regimen.

What to Look for When Purchasing Resistance Bands

Regardless of where you buy your resistance bands, there are a few crucial elements to consider to guarantee you obtain the correct product:

❖ *Resistance Level:* Resistance bands come in three different resistance levels: light, medium, and heavy. As a senior, you should choose a band that provides enough resistance to challenge your muscles without straining your joints or causing injury. Beginners should start with a light or medium band and develop as their strength grows.

❖ *Durability:* Look for bands made of high-quality natural latex or synthetics. The thicker and more sturdy the band, the longer it will endure and be less likely to snap or rip while in use. While thinner, cheaper bands may appear appealing, investing in a higher-quality device ensures safety and longevity.

❖ *Length and Width:* Consider the length and width of the band based on the workouts you intend to perform. Longer bands are more versatile and may be utilized for a larger range of activities, whilst shorter loops are better suited for lower body workouts like side steps and clamshells.

❖ *Grip and Comfort:* Some resistance bands include handles or fabric coverings, which can improve grip and lessen discomfort during use. This is especially useful for seniors with arthritis or those who may have difficulty gripping a basic latex band.

Finally, resistance bands are available in a variety of locations, including online and in-store. Whether you want a simple buy from a local retailer or a higher-end one from a specialist fitness company, there are numerous options to meet your fitness objectives and budget. By choosing the correct bands, you can position yourself for success as you try to increase your strength, mobility, and general health.

Safety Tips For Using Resistance Bands

Prioritize safety when training with any fitness equipment to avoid injuries and ensure a great experience. Here are detailed safety recommendations to consider when using resistance bands:

1. Select the appropriate resistance band for your fitness level

The first and most crucial safety recommendation is to choose a resistance band that is appropriate for your current fitness level. Resistance bands are graded as mild, medium, heavy, and very heavy. Each color usually correlates to a specific resistance level, however this can differ depending on the manufacturer, so always check the product's packing or instructions.

For beginners, it's best to start with a light resistance band so you can do exercises with perfect form and control.
Intermediate and advanced users can proceed to medium or heavy bands as they gain strength and confidence.

Using a too-powerful band can lead to poor form, strain, or even damage, particularly in seniors. It's always a good idea to start with lower resistance and gradually raise the intensity as your muscles adjust.

2. Inspect the Resistance Bands Regularly for Wear and Tear

Before beginning any workout, check your resistance bands for signs of wear and tear. Resistance bands are often made of latex or rubber, which can deteriorate over time, particularly if used frequently or stored improperly.

Watch out for:
  - ➤ *Cracks or Splits in the substance*
  - ➤ *Thinning parts of the band*
  - ➤ *Discoloration or unexpected changes in texture.*

If you observe any of these symptoms, replace the band immediately to reduce the danger of it snapping while in use. A sudden breakage while exercising might result in harm, especially to the face or joints.

3. Secure the band properly before each exercise

To avoid mishaps, the resistance band must be properly secured. Depending on the activity, you may need to anchor the band to a solid object or fasten it beneath your feet. Make sure whatever you're using to anchor the band is strong and stable.

For example, when performing standing exercises with the band looped beneath your feet, ensure that it is evenly placed and that there is no slack, as this could cause instability throughout the activity. If you're anchoring the band to a door, make sure it's closed and latched and put the anchor point at the appropriate height for the exercise you're doing.

4. Maintain the proper form and posture

Maintaining proper form and posture is critical for both safety and efficacy when using resistance bands. Because these bands create stress, it's tempting to let them drag your body into a compromised position, which might strain muscles or joints.

Controlled movements should be used throughout the workout, from the beginning to the end. Never allow the band to snap back unexpectedly, as this can result in harm.
Engage your core muscles throughout each action to protect your lower back and enhance overall balance.
If you're doing standing workouts, make sure your feet are properly positioned and shoulder width apart. When sitting, maintain an upright posture and, if required, support your back.

5. Begin slowly and build gradually

Seniors who are new to resistance bands or fitness, in general, should start carefully and progressively increase the intensity of their routines. Begin with simple workouts with low resistance and focus on fewer repetitions.

Once you're comfortable and confident in your motions, you can raise the amount of repetitions or the resistance of the band. Rushing into high-resistance exercises can cause muscle tension, pain, and even damage. By gradually introducing new motions, you allow your muscles and joints to adapt, building both strength and endurance over time.

6. Avoid overstretching the band

It may be tempting to extend the resistance band to its maximum capacity to get the most out of your workout, but overstretching can dramatically increase your risk of injury. Most resistance bands should only be stretched two to three times their resting length.

When you overstretch the band:
  - ➢ *It places undue tension on your muscles and joints, increasing the likelihood of strains and sprains.*
  - ➢ *The band is more susceptible to snap, which can result in a sudden injury.*
  - ➢ *Your range of motion may be compromised, resulting in poor form and technique.*

To avoid overstretching, use gradual and controlled movements and never draw the band to its maximum limit.

7. Breathe properly during the workout

Proper breathing is frequently forgotten during resistance band workouts, yet it is crucial for preserving safety and increasing the efficacy of your workout. Holding your breath, especially during strength activities, can create excessive strain in your body and induce dizziness or fainting.

> ➤ *Exhale throughout the exercise's exertion phase, which occurs when you draw or push the band.*
> ➤ *Inhale as you return to the starting position, giving your body a moment to rest before the next repetition.*

Breathing correctly regulates your heart rate, keeps a consistent supply of oxygen to your muscles, and lowers the risk of overexertion, especially for seniors who may have respiratory or cardiovascular issues.

8. Modify exercises according to mobility and fitness levels

Not all exercises are appropriate for everyone, particularly seniors with limited mobility or certain health issues. Resistance band exercises are easily adaptable to suit different fitness levels or physical restrictions.

> ➤ *If standing exercises become too difficult, move to sitting alternatives that offer additional support and stability.*

> *If an activity produces pain or discomfort, stop right away and alter the movement or resistance level.*
> *Consult with a physical therapist or personal trainer who specializes in senior fitness to ensure that the activities you select are appropriate for your specific needs.*

By tailoring exercises to your ability, you can limit the chance of injury while still getting the benefits of resistance band training.

9. Cool down and stretch after your workout

After your resistance band workout, you should cool down and stretch your muscles to enhance recovery and flexibility. Use the resistance bands to help with gentle stretches, concentrating on the regions addressed throughout the exercise session.

Cooling down helps to minimize muscle stiffness, enhance circulation, and return your heart rate to normal. Stretching after a workout can also reduce muscle discomfort and maintain joint flexibility, which is especially important for seniors.

10. Listen to your body and rest as needed

Finally, always listen to your body and rest as needed. Overworking your muscles without enough rest can cause fatigue, an increased risk of injury, and delayed recovery times.

If you feel pain during an activity, you should stop immediately and analyze if you're utilizing the proper technique, and resistance level, or are overexerting yourself. Pain is your body's way of telling you something is wrong, and pushing through it can cause long-term damage.

Resting between workouts allows your muscles to recuperate and strengthen, which is essential for maintaining long-term strength and mobility as you age.

Incorporating these safety measures into your resistance band workouts can help you exercise more successfully while reducing the danger of injury. Always take your time, practice perfect form, and select activities that are appropriate for your fitness level.

Creating A Comfortable Workout Space

Creating a dedicated, pleasant training environment is critical to sustaining a consistent and enjoyable exercise regimen, especially for seniors over 70. A well-organized and safe atmosphere can improve the effectiveness of your workouts, lower the chance of injury, and make exercising a pleasant and stress-free experience. *Here's a step-by-step approach to creating a workout area that encourages frequent use while also supporting your health and fitness goals.*

1. Choosing the Right Location

The first step in creating a workout room is determining the best location in your home. You don't need a vast room; even a tiny, devoted nook can be converted into a practical space for resistance band activities. Ideally, the room should possess the following characteristics:

- ❖ *Good ventilation:* Exercising in a stuffy environment can be difficult, especially during vigorous activity. Ensure that there is enough airflow in the room by opening windows or utilizing fans.
- ❖ *Natural light:* Natural sunlight not only improves mood and vitality but also makes the environment more inviting. If feasible, find a location near a window to receive natural

light. If that's not an option, make sure the area is well-lit to avoid accidents.

❖ *Peaceful and private:* Distractions can distract your concentration, so choose a peaceful location away from the main flow of your home. You don't need a completely isolated environment, but locating a place with few distractions will help you concentrate.

2. Flooring Considerations

The type of flooring in your training environment is critical to both safety and comfort. Hard surfaces, such as tile, wood, or concrete, can be difficult on your joints, particularly during standing workouts. Consider the following solutions for increased support and cushioning:

❖ *Exercise mats:* A comfortable, non-slip exercise mat can make a significant difference when practicing standing or sitting resistance band exercises. Mats cushion your joints and lessen the chance of slipping, making them an excellent addition to your area.

❖ *Carpeted areas:* If your home has carpeted floors, it can provide extra cushioning; however, the surface should not be overly thick or uneven, as this can interfere with your balance. A thinner, more sturdy carpet performs well, especially when combined with a mat for specialized activities.

3. Decluttering and Safety First

A clutter-free environment is essential for a safe and effective workout area. This is especially true for elders, as tripping hazards and impediments can result in damage. *Here are some safety things to consider:*

* ❖ *Clear the area of obstacles:* Remove any furniture, rugs, or loose items from the training area that may cause trips or falls. Make sure there is enough area to move freely, especially for workouts that require standing, walking, or balancing.
* ❖ *Sturdy furniture for support:* While you'll be utilizing resistance bands for most of your exercises, keeping a sturdy chair or table nearby can provide extra support as needed. For sitting workouts, be sure the chair is stable and does not slip or tip over easily.
* ❖ *Adequate space for movement:* Make sure you have adequate space around you to completely stretch your arms and legs. Resistance band exercises sometimes need wide motions, so having enough space will allow you to do each exercise with the appropriate form.

4. Essential Equipment and Tools

Setting up a workout environment for resistance band workouts does not require a lot of fancy equipment, but having a few key things will improve your comfort and convenience:

❖ Naturally, resistance bands are the focal point of your workout gear. Make sure you have a range of bands with varied tension levels (low, medium, and heavy) to accommodate your fitness improvement. To keep them organized, place them in a nearby basket or drawer that is easily accessible.

❖ Many resistance band programs for seniors include seated exercises, so a solid, comfortable chair is important. Choose a chair with a straight back and no armrests to ensure a wide range of motion during workouts.

❖ Some exercises necessitate securing the resistance band to a solid surface. Wall anchors and door attachments are handy ways to safely secure your bands at various heights. Make sure these attachments are securely fastened and can withstand the tension from the bands.

To aid with post-workout recuperation, keep a foam roller or massage ball accessible. These gadgets can help to relieve muscle tension and prevent pain after a workout.

5. Comfortable temperature settings

It is critical to keep your workout area at a comfortable temperature. Extreme temperatures can have an impact on your performance and motivation, so make sure the environment is pleasant and not too hot or cold. Maintaining a normal room temperature is especially important for elders since it reduces strain on the cardiovascular system.

Set the room temperature to a comfortable level before beginning your workout. If the room does not have a naturally comfortable climate, fans, space heaters, or portable air conditioners can help manage the temperature.

6. Incorporating visual cues for motivation

Making your training room visually appealing might help you stay motivated and thrilled to exercise regularly. Here are some tips for building a welcoming and motivating environment:

❖ *Inspiring quotations or posters:* Place motivational quotes or posters on your walls to remind you of your fitness goals. Positive affirmations can motivate you to stay on track and overcome any problems.

❖ *Plants and greenery:* Bringing nature indoors with houseplants may create a relaxing and pleasant atmosphere. According to research, greenery reduces stress and improves mood, making your training room more relaxing.

❖ *Mirrors:* Installing a mirror in your training area will allow you to evaluate your form and posture during activities. It also helps to make the environment feel wider and more open, which is very useful when working in a small location.

7. Music or Audio Support

Many people believe that music improves their workout experience by offering an energy boost or a peaceful background, depending on the sort of exercise. Soothing music or guided audio programs can help seniors enjoy their workouts while also improving time and rhythm.

Set up a small speaker or use wireless headphones to listen to your favorite music or workout videos. Choose music that matches the tempo and intensity of your workout to help you stay focused and motivated.

8. Storage Solutions That Are Accessible

Having a designated area to put your training equipment in keeps your space neat and organized. Easy access to your gear also increases your chances of sticking to your program.

Storage containers, baskets, or shelves are ideal for storing resistance bands, water bottles, and other equipment. This keeps your workout environment tidy and helps to avoid misplaced materials.

Always keep a towel and water bottle within arm's reach. Staying hydrated is essential for retaining energy throughout your workout, and a towel will keep you comfy during longer sessions.

By taking the time to create a pleasant, organized, and safe workout environment, you can support your fitness goals while also improving your overall health. For seniors over 70, this can make all the difference in maintaining consistency, keeping motivated, and reaping the benefits of regular exercise. A well-designed room that considers safety, convenience, and comfort will allow you to get the most out of your resistance band workouts and ensure long-term fitness success.

CHAPTER 3: PREPARING YOUR BODY FOR EXERCISE

The Value Of Warm-Up Routines For Seniors

As we age, our bodies naturally change, affecting how we move and react to physical exercise. Seniors above the age of 70 may have diminished flexibility, muscular mass, slower reaction times, and tightened joints. These changes can make physical activity more difficult and, without sufficient preparation, increase the risk of injury.

A warm-up regimen is thus necessary for seniors, acting as a solid basis before engaging in any sort of exercise, including low-impact exercises such as resistance band training. Below, we'll look at the significance of warm-up exercises for seniors, highlighting the multiple benefits they give for overall health, mobility, and injury prevention.

1. Improves blood flow and circulation

One of the most important goals of any warm-up is to progressively enhance blood flow to the muscles. This process is especially crucial for elders because circulation can become less effective with aging. The heart pumps slower, and blood arteries may become less elastic, resulting in decreased oxygen supply to muscles and tissues.

A proper warm-up helps to "wake up" the cardiovascular system by gradually raising the heart rate and improving circulation. This increase in blood flow guarantees that muscles receive more oxygen and nutrients, allowing them to perform well during exercise. Improved circulation also promotes joint lubrication, which is especially advantageous for seniors suffering from arthritis or joint stiffness.

2. Improves flexibility and range of motion

Flexibility decreases with age, making it more difficult for seniors to accomplish daily activities that demand a wide range of motion, such as reaching overhead, bending down, or rotating from side to side. A well-planned warm-up exercise can help to overcome these restrictions by relaxing muscles and enhancing joint mobility.

Warm-up activities help seniors stretch their muscles and develop their flexibility by using slow, controlled motions. This improves overall movement and reduces the chance of damage during more intensive exercises. Exercises like arm circles, leg swings, and shoulder rolls, for example, can assist in releasing stiff muscles and enhance mobility in important areas like the shoulders, hips, and back.

3. Reduces the risk of injury

One of the most serious concerns for seniors who participate in physical activity is the risk of injury. The body's vulnerability to strains, sprains, and other injuries increases with age, especially when muscles and joints are cold or tight. Warming up appropriately reduces this danger by progressively preparing the body for exercise.

When muscles are cold, they become less flexible and more prone to tearing or straining. A warm-up routine increases muscle temperature, making them more flexible and less prone to injury. A warm-up also helps to engage the neurological system, improving coordination and reaction speeds, which are critical for avoiding falls or unexpected movements that could cause damage.

This is especially crucial for seniors, as the recuperation process slows as they age. Warm-up exercises can help older persons reduce their risk of injury while also allowing them to exercise safely and consistently.

4. It prepares the body and mind for physical activity

Warm-up routines prepare the body physically and emotionally. Light, repetitive movements before a workout assist seniors adjust their concentration, becoming more in tune with their bodies and mindful of their emotions. This mental preparation is vital for elders because it promotes mindfulness during exercise and can help prevent overexertion.

Seniors, for example, might measure their energy levels and identify stiffness or soreness in their muscles and joints by beginning with easy breathing exercises or light stretching. This increased awareness enables individuals to alter their training as needed, selecting routines that are appropriate for their present physical state.

The mental part of warming up helps seniors gain confidence in their abilities to move safely and pleasantly. By gradually introducing exercise, individuals are less likely to feel overwhelmed or nervous about their workout, resulting in a joyful and empowering exercise experience.

5. Promotes joint health and longevity

Many senior citizens feel joint discomfort or stiffness, particularly in the knees, hips, and shoulders. Conditions like osteoarthritis, which causes cartilage in joints to break down over time, can exacerbate joint difficulties. Without sufficient care and preparation, these joints may be more prone to injury or degradation.

Warm-up activities are especially beneficial to joint health because they increase the production of synovial fluid. This fluid functions as a lubricant, reducing friction between bones and making joints move more easily. Regular warm-up activities can help seniors protect their joints, reduce discomfort, and increase their general range of motion.

Low-impact warm-up motions such as seated stretches, modest leg raises, or controlled arm movements might help seniors with arthritis or other joint difficulties relieve stiffness and pain, allowing them to exercise without difficulty.

6. Promotes muscle activation and engagement

As we age, our muscles become less sensitive, and seniors may find it more difficult to engage certain muscle groups properly. This can result in muscular imbalances, with some muscles overused and others underutilized. Muscle imbalances can raise the risk of injury while limiting overall strength and mobility.

A warm-up routine activates the primary muscle groups that will be used during the workout, ensuring that they are adequately engaged and prepared to perform. Leg swings, arm circles, and moderate squats are examples of exercises that might help seniors develop a more balanced, coordinated movement pattern.

By stimulating these muscles before exercise, seniors can increase their overall performance and get the most out of their activity. This not only increases strength but also ensures that the correct muscles are working together, lowering the risk of overuse problems.

7. Improves coordination and balance

Balance and coordination tend to deteriorate with age, increasing the risk of falls and accidents, which are the major causes of injury among the elderly. Incorporating balance-focused warm-up activities can help older persons improve their stability and coordination, lowering the risk of falling.

Exercises like single-leg stand, heel-to-toe walking, and modest weight shifts can help seniors practice keeping their balance in a controlled manner. These warm-up activities improve the body's proprioception—the sensation of where it is in space—allowing seniors to move more confidently and steadily during their workout.

Warm-ups improve balance, which leads to greater performance in regular activities including walking, climbing stairs, and standing from a seated position.

8. Supports cardiovascular health

Warm-up routines that include light aerobic workouts, such as marching in place, arm swings, or gentle walking, can help improve cardiovascular health. These activities progressively increase the heart rate, which improves cardiac function and circulation. Maintaining cardiovascular health is critical for seniors' general well-being since it helps prevent illnesses like heart disease, high blood pressure, and stroke.

Seniors can boost their cardiovascular system by gradually increasing their heart rate during warm-up exercises. This prepares children for more demanding exercises and promotes long-term heart health.

For seniors over 70, the significance of a proper warm-up routine cannot be emphasized. Warming up is vital for preparing the body and mind for exercise, as it improves circulation and flexibility, lowers the chance of injury, and supports joint health. Seniors who incorporate a well-structured warm-up into their routine will be more active, healthier, and confident in their abilities to move safely and effectively, boosting long-term strength, mobility, and independence.

Simple Stretching And Mobility Exercises With Resistance Bands

Stretching and mobility exercises are essential components of any fitness plan, especially for seniors over 70. These exercises serve to maintain flexibility, reduce stiffness, increase range of motion, and prevent injury. Stretching can be more successful when combined with resistance bands, allowing you to target muscles and joints more precisely while also moderately building strength. Resistance bands are a low-impact, adjustable solution that can help seniors increase their mobility while remaining safe.

In this part, we'll look at simple stretching and mobility exercises that seniors can do with resistance bands. These exercises are intended to be moderate but effective, catering to a variety of fitness levels while focusing on certain regions of the body.

Benefits of Stretching with Resistance Bands

Stretching helps to relieve muscle tension, increasing mobility and lowering discomfort, particularly in tight areas like the back, hips, shoulders, and legs. For seniors, the combination of stretching and resistance bands provides various benefits:

❖ Resistance bands create regulated tension, allowing muscles to extend deeper than static stretching alone.
❖ Regular stretching with bands improves flexibility, making daily actions like bending, reaching, and turning simpler.
❖ Stretching with resistance bands promotes good posture by targeting the muscles that support the spine and shoulders.
❖ Resistance bands allow for moderate tension increases, making movement easier to manage and avoiding overstretching or muscular strain.

Warm up your body before beginning any stretching routine. Walking, moving in steps, or doing small arm swings can all help to promote circulation and prepare the muscles for more focused stretches. Once warmed up, seniors can begin stretching and mobility exercises with resistance bands.

1. Seated Hamstring Stretch

The hamstrings, which are located in the rear of the thighs, are necessary for walking and other lower-body activities. Stretching the hamstrings can help reduce stress in the lower back and legs.

How to perform:

1. Sit on the floor or in a solid chair, legs extended in front of you.
2. Loop the resistance band around the ball of one foot, gripping the ends with both hands.
3. Keep your back straight and gradually draw the band toward you, maintaining your leg straight. You should feel a stretch in the back of your leg.
4. Hold for 20-30 seconds, then switch to the opposite leg.

This exercise softly extends the hamstrings while the band offers light resistance, allowing you to manage the stretch and avoid damage.

2. Chest Opener Stretch

The chest opening stretch works the pectoral muscles and improves posture by counteracting the forward rounding of the shoulders. This stretch is very useful for seniors who spend a lot of time sitting.

How to perform:

1. Stand or sit with your feet shoulder-width apart.
2. Hold the resistance band behind your back, with both hands about shoulder-width apart.
3. Gently pull the band outward while straightening your arms, expanding your chest, and bringing your shoulder blades together.
4. Hold the stretch for 15-20 seconds before relaxing and repeating.

This stretch relaxes tight chest muscles and strengthens the upper back, which can lead to improved posture and less back pain.

3. Seated Shoulder Stretch

This exercise focuses on the shoulders and upper back, helping to develop flexibility in these areas, which are essential for everyday actions like reaching and lifting.

How to perform:

1. Sit comfortably in a chair, feet flat on the floor.
2. Hold the resistance band in both hands and stretch your arms in front of you at shoulder height.

3. Gently draw the band outward until your arms are fully stretched to the sides while keeping your shoulders relaxed.
4. Hold for 20 seconds before slowly returning to the start position and repeating.

This stretch, which includes a resistance band, promotes more active muscle engagement, resulting in greater shoulder flexibility and less stiffness.

4. Standing Calf Stretch

Calf muscles are typically disregarded, yet stretching them can increase ankle mobility and lower the risk of falling.

How to perform:

1. Stand with your feet hip-width apart, then loop the resistance band around the ball of one foot.
2. Step back slightly with the opposite foot, keeping your front leg straight and your heel on the ground.
3. Pull gently on the band to enhance the strain in your calf.
4. Hold the posture for 20-30 seconds, then switch to the opposite leg.

This stretch promotes flexibility in the calves and Achilles tendon, which is necessary for walking and balance.

5. Seated Hip Stretch

This exercise is designed to gently stretch and develop the hip muscles, which are essential for balance and movement.

How to perform:

1. Sit on a chair, with both feet flat on the floor.
2. Loop the resistance band around your thighs, slightly above the knees.
3. Slowly press your knees outwards to stretch the band.
4. Hold for 10 seconds before slowly releasing and repeating.

This stretch opens up the hips, increases flexibility, and promotes greater balance.

6. Quadriceps Stretch

Walking, standing, and sitting all rely heavily on the quadriceps. This stretch promotes flexibility in these critical muscles.

How to perform:

1. Sit in a chair, one leg out in front of you.
2. Wrap the resistance band around the ankle of the extended leg.
3. Gently pull the band, bringing your heel closer to your torso while keeping your back straight.

4. Hold the stretch for 20-30 seconds before switching to the other leg.

This exercise gently stretches the quadriceps, while the resistance band adds controlled strain.

7. Upper Back Stretch

This exercise works the muscles between the shoulder blades, relieving tension and improving posture.

How to perform:

1. Sit or stand with your feet shoulder-width apart.
2. Hold the resistance band in front of you with both hands, shoulder-width apart.
3. Pull the band outwards, keeping your arms at shoulder height and your shoulders down.
4. Hold the stretch for 15-20 seconds before relaxing and repeating.

This exercise, which stretches the upper back, can help to relieve shoulder and neck stiffness and pain.

8. Seated Triceps Stretch

This stretch focuses on the triceps, the muscles on the back of your arms, which helps to enhance flexibility and range of motion.

How to perform:

1. Sit on a chair, feet flat on the floor.
2. Hold the resistance band with one hand and place it behind your back.
3. Using your other hand, slowly pull the band upward, stretching the triceps behind your back.
4. Hold for 20-30 seconds and then switch arms.

This stretch is a mild technique to enhance arm flexibility, which is useful for actions like lifting and reaching.

Incorporating resistance bands into stretching and mobility exercises can offer seniors a safe, effective, and gentle way to maintain flexibility and enhance joint health. These exercises not only relieve stiffness but also improve balance and mobility, making daily tasks easier and fostering independence. Seniors who execute these basic stretches regularly can benefit from increased range of motion, better posture, and increased strength, all of which contribute to a healthier and more active lifestyle.

How To Avoid Muscle Strain And Injury

Preventing muscular strain and injury is an important part of any workout regimen, especially for seniors over 70, who are more prone to such problems due to age-related changes in muscle mass, flexibility, and joint stability. Seniors can safely engage in resistance band exercises and other forms of physical activity if they take a proactive attitude and follow specific instructions.

The following is a detailed guide on preventing muscle strain and injury, specifically in the context of resistance band exercises for seniors.

1. Understand Your Body's Limits

Recognizing your body's limitations is a critical strategy for reducing muscle strain. As we age, our muscles, tendons, and ligaments naturally lose flexibility, making them more vulnerable to damage. This means that pushing your body too hard or attempting to execute exercises above your present fitness level can cause muscle strain, sprains, or even more serious injuries such as tears.

> ➤ *Start Slow: Whether you are a beginner or have some expertise, always begin with workouts that are appropriate for your current fitness level. Seniors who are new to resistance band workouts should begin with low-resistance*

bands and easy routines. Avoid attempting advanced exercises before understanding the fundamentals.

➢ **Listen to Your Body:** *Pay attention to any discomfort or pain when exercising. Muscle soreness is typical, particularly after new or strenuous activities, but strong or sudden pain indicates that something is wrong. If you experience discomfort when exercising, stop immediately, analyze the situation, and avoid pushing through the pain to prevent further injury.*

2. Focus on proper warm-up and stretching

Warming up before an exercise is one of the most efficient techniques to avoid muscle strain and damage. A good warm-up routine gets the body ready for more intensive physical activity by increasing blood flow to the muscles, enhancing flexibility, and gradually stimulating the joints and tendons.

➢ **Dynamic Stretching:** *Before beginning resistance band exercises, perform dynamic stretches to improve your range of motion and lower your chance of injury. These include modest, regulated movements that correspond to the workout you're about to conduct. Leg swings and arm circles, for example, can aid in the relaxation of important muscle groups and joints.*

➤ *Band-Assisted Warm-Ups: Resistance bands can be used during warm-ups to target specific muscle groups. Begin with gentle stretches and motions with the band, focusing on the shoulders, back, hips, and legs. Stretching with a resistance band can help you warm up and stretch your muscles without overworking them.*

3. Use the proper form and technique

One of the most common causes of muscular tension is incorrect exercise form. Maintaining good technique, especially when using resistance bands, is critical to ensuring that the relevant muscles are targeted and strain is distributed properly.

➤ *Posture: Maintain appropriate posture throughout the exercises. This entails standing straight, keeping your core engaged, and shoulders back, and avoiding slouching or hunching over. Good posture not only prevents injury but also increases the efficacy of the activity.*

➤ *Controlled Movements: Avoid jerky or quick movements, which can put too much strain on your muscles and joints. Instead, go for gradual, controlled motions that allow the muscles to fully engage and limit the risk of damage. For example, when performing a banded pull-apart, move carefully and concentrate on tightening the muscles at the top of the action.*

➢ **Breathing:** *Proper breathing techniques can also help prevent injuries. Inhale at the less strenuous portion of the exercise, and exhale during the exertion. This keeps oxygen flowing to your muscles, lowering the risk of overexertion.*

4. Gradually increase resistance

While it may be tempting to increase the resistance level of your bands to see faster results, doing so too quickly increases the risk of muscle strain. Progression is vital in any workout plan, but it must be done cautiously and gradually.

➢ **Start with Low Resistance:** *If you're new to resistance band exercises, start with the lowest resistance possible and work your way up. As your strength grows, you can progressively raise the resistance of the bands, but be aware of how your body reacts. It is preferable to do an activity with a lighter band and proper form than to fight with a bigger band and risk injury.*

➢ **Increase Repetitions Before Resistance:** *To avoid damage, increase repetitions before increasing resistance. Begin by performing more repetitions of a certain exercise using a lighter band. Once your muscles have acclimated and you can comfortably complete the exercises, you can start increasing the resistance.*

5. Rest and Recovery

Recovery is often disregarded, although it is an important part of injury prevention. Allowing your muscles to rest between workouts allows them to recover and strengthen, reducing strain.

> *Allow Time for Muscle Repair: It is especially crucial for elders to avoid training the same muscle groups on consecutive days. If you undertake an upper-body resistance band workout one day, allow those muscles to heal by focusing on your lower body or taking a day off.*

> *Incorporate Rest Days: Even if you believe you can exercise every day, rest days are essential for avoiding overuse problems. Overworking your muscles without proper rest can result in injuries and long-term damage.*

> *Post-Workout Stretching: After each workout, perform static stretches to help cool down your muscles and increase flexibility. Resistance band stretches can also help lengthen tight muscles and promote relaxation after exercise.*

6. Hydration and Nutrition

Staying hydrated and eating properly is another important component in avoiding muscle strain and injury. Dehydration can cause muscle cramps and limit your body's capacity to recuperate from exercise.

➤ **Stay Hydrated:** *Drink water prior to, during, and following your workout. Muscles are made up of 75% water, thus staying hydrated helps them operate properly.*

➤ **Consume a Balanced Diet:** *A diet high in protein, healthy fats, and carbohydrates supports muscle repair and recovery. Seniors should focus on ingesting enough protein to promote muscular preservation, as aging can naturally cause muscle loss.*

7. Know when to stop and seek professional advice

Finally, understanding when to stop is critical to avoiding major harm. If you have prolonged pain or discomfort while exercising, consult a doctor or physical therapist. They can assist in discovering underlying problems and advise on safe exercises or changes.

If you have pain in specific joints or muscles, tailor the workout to your ability. Resistance band exercises are very flexible, so you can change the range of motion or lower the resistance to make the workout more bearable.

Understanding your body's limitations, focusing on good warm-up and stretching, utilizing proper form and technique, gradually increasing resistance, allowing for adequate rest, and paying attention to hydration and nutrition can all help lower your risk of muscular strain and injury. Seniors over the age of 70 can safely perform resistance band exercises and reap the benefits of increased strength, balance, and mobility without jeopardizing their health.

Preventing muscle strain and injury involves both awareness and discipline, but with the appropriate technique, seniors can stay active and healthy well into their golden years.

CHAPTER 4: RESISTANCE BAND
EXERCISES FOR BEGINNERS

1. Pull Chest Apart

Instructions:

1. Stand with your feet shoulder-width apart, holding the resistance band in front of you at chest level with both hands.
2. Keep your arms straight and pull the band apart with your hands outward until they are fully extended to the sides.
3. Slowly return to your starting position, keeping control of the band throughout.

Benefits:

- Enhances posture by strengthening the upper back and shoulder muscles.
- Increases shoulder mobility, lowering the likelihood of injury during everyday tasks.

2. Lat Pulldown

Instructions:

1. Secure the band above you (for example, to a doorframe or a high anchor).
2. Sit or stand holding the band in both hands, arms stretched overhead.
3. Pull the band down to your chest, keeping your back straight and your elbows sliding down and back.
4. Slowly return to your starting location.

Benefits:

- Strengthens the lats, assisting in daily pulling motions.
- Improves core stability by exercising abdominal muscles throughout the activity.

3. Seated Row

Instructions:

1. Sit with your legs extended, loop the band over your feet, and grip the ends in both hands.
2. Keep your back straight and draw the band towards your torso, bringing your elbows close to your sides.
3. Slowly return to the starting position.

Benefits:

- Increases upper back strength, improves posture and relieves back discomfort.
- Engages core muscles, which improves balance and stability.

4. Pallof Press

Instructions:

1. Secure the band to a stable item at chest level.
2. Stand sideways to the anchor, clutching the band with both hands to your chest.
3. Press your arms straight out in front of you, fighting the band's pull, then return to the beginning position.

Benefits:

- Develops core strength by preventing rotation and increasing balance.
- Strengthens the oblique muscles, improving overall body stability.

5. Band Side Step

Instructions:

1. Put a resistance band around your legs, right above the knees.
2. Stand with your feet hip-width apart, slightly bend your knees, and take a step to the side while keeping tension in the band.
3. Return to the original place and repeat on the other side.

Benefits:

- Activates hip abductors, which lowers the chance of knee injury.
- Improves lateral movement, which is necessary for everyday activities such as walking and balance.

6. Clam shell

Instructions:

1. Lie on your side, knees bent and a resistance band wrapped over your thighs.
2. Keep your feet together and elevate your upper knee while your hips remain solid.
3. Slowly lower your knee down and repeat.

Benefits:

- Strengthens the glutes, improving hip stability and minimizing lower back pain.
- Improves pelvic stability, which is important for balance and posture.

7. Side Leg Lift

Instructions:

1. Stand with the resistance band around your ankles, using a wall or chair for support.
2. Lift one leg to the side while keeping your body straight and your foot contracted.
3. Slowly return to your starting posture and switch legs.

Benefits:

- Strengthens the hip and glute muscles, which improves balance and stability.
- Improves lateral mobility, which is essential for walking and preventing falls.

8. Chest Press

Instructions:

1. Secure the band behind you (for example, around a solid object or a door).
2. Hold the band at chest height with both hands and stretch your arms forward until completely extended.
3. Slowly return to the beginning posture while keeping your back straight and core engaged.

Benefits:

- Increases chest and shoulder strength, enhancing upper-body function.
- Engages the core, improving posture and stability.

CHAPTER 5: RESISTANCE BAND EXERCISES FOR INTERMEDIATES

1. Hip Thrust

Instructions:

1. Sit with your upper back resting on a bench, knees bent, feet flat on the floor.
2. Place a resistance band above your knees.
3. Drive your hips upward, squeezing your glutes at the top.
4. Slowly lower your hips back down and repeat.

Benefits:

- Builds stronger glutes and hamstrings, improving posture and reducing lower back pain.
- Enhances athletic performance by improving hip extension power, useful for walking and climbing stairs.

2. Bulgarian Split Squat

Instructions:

1. Stand facing away from a bench, placing one foot on the bench behind you.
2. Hold a resistance band under your front foot, gripping the handles.
3. Lower into a squat, keeping your front knee aligned with your toes.
4. Push back up, maintaining balance.

Benefits:

- Strengthens legs and glutes while improving single-leg balance.
- Increases mobility and stability, reducing the risk of falls.

3. Pull Down

Instructions:

1. Attach the band to a high point.
2. Stand and grip the band with both hands.
3. Pull the band down toward your chest, squeezing your shoulder blades together.
4. Slowly release to the starting position.

Benefits:

- Strengthens upper back and shoulders, improving posture.
- Engages core muscles, supporting spinal health.

4. Banded Push-Up

Instructions:

1. Loop a resistance band around your upper back, holding the ends under your palms.
2. Perform a standard push-up, lowering your chest to the floor.
3. Push back up while resisting the band's tension.

Benefits:

- Strengthens chest, shoulders, and triceps.
- Improves core stability and upper body strength.

5. One Arm Shoulder Press

Instructions:

1. Step on the band with one foot, holding the other end in one hand at shoulder height.
2. Press the band upward until your arm is fully extended.
3. Slowly lower and repeat.

Benefits:

- Enhances shoulder stability and strength.
- Targets the deltoids, improving upper body function.

6. One Arm Row

Instructions:

1. Anchor the band at a low point.
2. Hold one end of the band and step back to create tension.
3. Pull the band toward your hip, squeezing your back muscles.
4. Release slowly.

Benefits:

- Strengthens the upper back and biceps.
- Improves posture and reduces back strain.

7. Bend Over

Instructions:

1. Stand on the band with feet shoulder-width apart, holding the ends in both hands.
2. Bend at the hips, keeping your back straight.

3. Pull the band upward, engaging your glutes and hamstrings, then lower.

Benefits:

- Engages the lower back, glutes, and hamstrings for improved strength.
- Helps prevent lower back pain by strengthening posterior chain muscles.

8. Banded Dead Bug

Instructions:

1. Lie on your back with knees bent, holding a resistance band above your head.
2. Lower one leg while pulling the opposite arm down, keeping tension in the band.
3. Return to the start and switch sides.

Benefits:

- Strengthens the core, improving balance and stability.
- Engages multiple muscle groups, enhancing coordination.

9. Banded Plank Walk

Instructions:

1. Place a resistance band around your wrists.
2. Get into a plank position, then step one hand to the side, followed by the other.
3. Repeat, alternating sides.

Benefits:

- Builds core strength and stability.
- Improves shoulder endurance and mobility.

CHAPTER 6: SEATED RESISTANCE BAND EXERCISES

---

1. Seated Pointed Toes (Calf Press)

Instructions:

1. Sit in a chair with your back straight.
2. Loop the resistance band under the ball of one foot, holding both ends of the band with your hands.
3. Extend your leg forward and point your toes toward the ceiling, then slowly point them downward.
4. Repeat for 10-15 reps, then switch legs.

Benefits:

- Strengthens calf muscles to support better walking and balance.
- Improves flexibility and range of motion in the ankles.

2. Seated Leg Lift

Instructions:

1. Sit up straight with your feet flat on the floor.
2. Loop the resistance band around one foot, holding both ends of the band.
3. Extend your leg out in front of you, lifting it until it's parallel to the floor.
4. Hold for 2-3 seconds, then slowly lower back down. Repeat 10-15 times and switch legs.

Benefits:

- Strengthens quadriceps and hip flexors, essential for leg mobility.
- Enhances knee stability, reducing the risk of injury.

3. Seated Leg Press

Instructions:

1. Sit with your back straight and loop a resistance band around the sole of one foot.
2. Hold both ends of the band and bend your knee towards you.
3. Straighten your leg by pushing against the band's resistance, then return to the bent position.
4. Repeat 10-15 times on each leg.

Benefits:

- Builds leg strength and stability for improved walking and standing.
- Helps maintain joint flexibility in the hips and knees.

4. Seated Hip Opening (Hip Abduction)

Instructions:

1. Sit in a chair with your feet flat on the floor.
2. Place a resistance band around your thighs just above the knees.
3. Slowly push your knees outward, stretching the band, and hold for 3-5 seconds.
4. Return to the starting position and repeat 10-15 times.

Benefits:

- Strengthens hip abductors for better balance and stability.
- Reduces the risk of falls by improving lateral movement.

5. Seated Abdominal Lean (Oblique Crunch)

Instructions:

1. Sit with a resistance band anchored securely under your feet.
2. Hold the ends of the band with both hands near your shoulders.
3. Slowly lean to one side while keeping your core engaged, then return to the center.
4. Repeat for the other side, alternating for 10-15 reps on each side.

Benefits:

- Strengthens oblique muscles for improved core stability.
- Enhances posture and reduces lower back strain.

6. Seated Chest Press

Instructions:

1. Sit upright with the resistance band anchored behind the chair.
2. Hold both ends of the band with your hands at chest level.
3. Press your arms forward, straightening them in front of you, then return to the start.
4. Repeat 10-15 times.

Benefits:

- Strengthens chest and arm muscles for improved upper body strength.
- Enhances posture by engaging chest and shoulder muscles.

CHAPTER 7: RESISTANCE BAND EXERCISES FOR ADVANCED LEVEL

1. Pull to Face (Resistance Band Face Pull)

Instructions:

1. Anchor the band at chest height.
2. Stand with feet shoulder-width apart and hold the band with both hands, arms extended in front of you.
3. Pull the band towards your face, keeping your elbows high and focusing on squeezing your shoulder blades together.
4. Pause briefly, then slowly return to the starting position.

Benefits:

- Improves posture by strengthening the rear delts and upper back muscles.
- Enhances shoulder stability by targeting the small rotator cuff muscles, which support shoulder joint health.

2. Front Squat

Instructions:

1. Stand on the resistance band with feet shoulder-width apart.
2. Hold the band handles at shoulder level, elbows bent.
3. Lower into a squat by bending at your hips and knees, keeping your chest up and knees tracking over your toes.
4. Push through your heels to return to the standing position.

Benefits:

- Builds lower body strength by engaging quadriceps, hamstrings, and glutes.
- Improves core stability as you maintain posture during the movement.

3. Single Leg Deadlift

Instructions:

1. Stand with one foot on the resistance band, holding both handles.
2. Hinge forward at the hips, extending your free leg behind you while lowering your torso.
3. Keep your back straight and shoulders level, then return to the standing position.

Benefits:

- Develops balance and stability by engaging core and leg muscles.
- Strengthens posterior chain (hamstrings, glutes, lower back) for better functional movement.

4. Bear Crawl with Resistance Band

Instructions:

1. Place the band around your waist and secure the other end to a stationary object.
2. Start in a bear crawl position with knees hovering slightly off the ground.
3. Crawl forward and backward, resisting the pull of the band, keeping your core tight.

Benefits:

- Engages the entire body with a focus on shoulders, core, and legs.
- Improves cardiovascular endurance as well as overall strength.

5. Chest Crossover

Instructions:

1. Anchor the band behind you at chest height.
2. Hold the handles with arms extended out to the sides.
3. Bring your hands together in front of you, crossing one arm over the other.
4. Slowly return to the starting position and alternate the crossing arm.

Benefits:

- Targets chest muscles effectively by working both the pectoralis major and minor.
- Improves shoulder mobility and flexibility as you cross the arms.

6. Resistance Crunch

Instructions:

1. Anchor the band above you.
2. Lie on your back with your knees bent and hold the band handles.
3. Perform a crunch by engaging your core, and pulling the band handles down towards your knees.
4. Slowly return to the starting position.

Benefits:

- Strengthens core muscles, particularly the rectus abdominis.
- Improves stability and posture by working the deep core muscles.

7. Lateral Raise

Instructions:

1. Stand on the resistance band with feet shoulder-width apart, holding the handles at your sides.
2. With a slight bend in your elbows, raise your arms out to the sides until they are parallel to the floor.
3. Lower them back down slowly.

Benefits:

- Strengthens the shoulder muscles, especially the deltoids.
- Improves shoulder stability and mobility, which is essential for daily activities and injury prevention.

CHAPTER 8: ROUNDING OFF WITH FULL-BODY EXERCISES

1. Standing Row

Instructions:

1. Secure the resistance band at chest height to a stable object.
2. Hold the handles or ends of the band in each hand, stepping back to create tension.
3. Stand with feet shoulder-width apart, keeping your chest up and core engaged.
4. Pull the band towards you, leading with your elbows and squeezing your shoulder blades together.
5. Slowly return to the starting position.

Benefits:

- Strengthens back muscles, particularly the lats and rhomboids.
- Improves posture by targeting muscles that support the spine.

2. Banded Push-Ups

Instructions:

1. Loop a resistance band across your upper back, holding the ends under each hand in a push-up position.
2. Keep your body in a straight line from head to heels.
3. Lower yourself down by bending your elbows until your chest is close to the ground.
4. Push back up to the starting position, maintaining tension in the band.

Benefits:

- Increases chest and triceps strength by adding resistance to a standard push-up.
- Enhances core stability by forcing you to engage your abs throughout the movement.

3. Core Rotations

Instructions:

1. Anchor a resistance band at chest height to a sturdy object.
2. Stand sideways to the anchor point, holding the band with both hands extended in front of you.
3. Rotate your torso away from the anchor while keeping your arms straight.

4. Slowly return to the starting position, resisting the pull of the band.

Benefits:

- Strengthens the obliques and core muscles, improving rotational power.
- Enhances stability and balance by engaging the entire core.

4. Biceps Curl

Instructions:

1. Stand on the middle of the resistance band with feet shoulder-width apart.
2. Hold the ends of the band with palms facing forward and elbows tucked into your sides.
3. Curl your hands toward your shoulders, keeping your elbows stationary.
4. Slowly lower back down to the starting position.

Benefits:

- Build strength in the biceps and forearms.
- Improves arm endurance and muscle tone.

5. Triceps Extension

Instructions:

1. Step on the middle of the resistance band with one foot, holding the handles or ends in both hands.
2. Raise your arms overhead, keeping your elbows close to your ears.
3. Extend your arms upward, straightening the elbows.
4. Slowly bend your arms back to the starting position.

Benefits:

- Strengthens the triceps, helping improve upper-arm definition.
- Enhances arm endurance and function in everyday tasks.

6. Banded Deceleration Lunges

Instructions:

1. Loop the resistance band around your waist and secure it to a fixed point behind you.
2. Step forward into a lunge, keeping tension in the band.
3. Push back to the standing position, using your glutes and legs to resist the pull of the band.

Benefits:

- Improves lower-body strength, particularly in the quads and glutes.
- Enhances stability and control during dynamic movements.

7. Shoulder Press

Instructions:

1. Stand on the band with feet shoulder-width apart, holding the ends or handles at shoulder height.
2. Press the band overhead, fully extending your arms.
3. Slowly lower the band back to shoulder height.

Benefits:

- Strengthens the shoulders and upper back.
- Improves upper-body stability and overhead strength.

8. X-Band Squat

Instructions:

1. Stand on the band with feet shoulder-width apart, crossing the band in front of your body to form an "X."
2. Hold the handles or ends of the band at hip level.
3. Squat down by bending at the hips and knees, keeping your back straight.
4. Stand back up, squeezing your glutes at the top.

Benefits:

- Strengthens the lower body, particularly the glutes, quads, and hamstrings.
- Enhances balance and coordination.

CHAPTER 9: STAYING MOTIVATED AND OVERCOMING CHALLENGES

Tips For Maintaining Consistency With Your Exercise Routine

Preserving a consistent exercise regimen, particularly for seniors over the age of 70, can be difficult, but it is critical for preserving health and wellness. Regular physical activity has several advantages, including increased strength, balance, flexibility, and mental health. *Here are some practical ways to help elders stick to their fitness programs.*

1. Set realistic goals

Setting realistic, achievable goals is critical for maintaining motivation. Instead of striving for dramatic changes, concentrate on little, incremental gains. For example, progressively increase the number of repetitions and duration of your workouts. This strategy not only helps to minimize damage but also gives you a sense of success, making it easier to continue involved.

SMART Goals: Consider using the SMART criterion while developing goals. Make sure your goals are specific, measurable, attainable, relevant, and time-bound. Instead of saying, "I want to exercise more," you may say, "I will perform resistance band exercises for 20 minutes, three times a week, for the next month."

2. Create a schedule

Consistency is sometimes a product of regularity. Create a regular fitness program that works with your daily activities. Whether you prefer morning, afternoon, or evening workouts, select a time that works best for you and stick to it.

Use a planner or calendar to schedule particular times for exercise, just like you would for an essential appointment. Consistency in timing can help to reinforce the habit.

3. Make It enjoyable

Incorporating enjoyment into your training program will dramatically boost adherence. Choose activities that you enjoy and find entertaining, such as resistance band workouts, nature walks, or group lessons.

Changing up your routine helps keep things interesting and intriguing. Try new exercises or change venues. For example, you might conduct some workouts in the living room, some outside in the garden, or attend a local fitness class.

4. Find a workout buddy

Exercising with a friend or family member can help boost motivation and accountability. A gym partner can help you stick to your schedule, make exercises more fun, and provide a social aspect to your exercise.

If possible, consider joining a senior-focused workout club or class. This not only provides company but also allows you to meet like-minded people who have similar goals.

5. Track your progress

Keeping track of your progress can be quite motivating. Record your workouts in a diary, app, or calendar, noting the exercises you did, the time it took, and how you felt afterward.

Recognize and celebrate tiny wins along the way, such as finishing a particular number of workouts or increasing the weights you can lift. This positive reinforcement can boost motivation and make you pleased with your achievements.

6. Listen to your body

While consistency is vital, it's also critical to listen to your body. Pay attention to how you feel before, during, and after your workout. If you feel pain or exhaustion, take a break and alter your workouts as needed.

Include rest days in your schedule. Recovery is essential, particularly as we age, to avoid injury and exhaustion. Plan at least one or two days of rest per week to allow your body to recover.

7. Stay flexible and adaptable

Life is unpredictable, and your schedule may not always allow for a complete workout. Maintain flexibility in your approach and be open to changing your routine as needed. If you skip a workout, don't be too hard on yourself; instead, try to get back on track as quickly as possible.

If you're short on time, consider "micro-workouts," which are shorter sessions lasting 10-15 minutes. These can be equally useful and help you maintain regularity without being overwhelmed.

8. Educate yourself

Understanding the benefits of your workout regimen will help you stay committed. Read publications, attend workshops, or talk to fitness specialists who specialize in senior fitness.

Understanding how exercises affect your health and well-being might drive you to stay to your plan. It could also help you find new exercises or techniques to try.

9. Focus on the benefits

Regularly remind yourself of the myriad benefits of keeping active. Consistent exercise has numerous benefits, including improved strength, balance, energy levels, and mood enhancement.

Remember that exercise is more than simply physical fitness. It can boost mood, alleviate anxiety and sadness, and improve general mental health. Keeping these benefits in mind might be an effective incentive.

10. Incorporate Mindfulness

Mindfulness methods, such as meditation or yoga, can help you focus and stay motivated while exercising. These activities can help reduce stress and improve your general attitude toward exercise.

Consider incorporating mindfulness into your workouts. Concentrate on your breathing, bodily sensations, and motions. This method can increase your enjoyment of exercise and foster a stronger connection to your physical health.

Staying consistent with a fitness routine, especially for seniors, necessitates preparation, motivation, and flexibility. Setting reasonable objectives, developing a timetable, enjoying your workouts, and listening to your body can help you develop a long-term routine that improves your health and well-being. Remember that the fitness journey is personal, and acknowledging your progress, no matter how tiny, can have a huge impact on your resolve to stay active. Accept the process and enjoy the countless benefits of being fit and healthy throughout your older years.

Working Around Common Obstacles: Pain, Fatigue, And A Lack Of Time

Regular exercise is essential for seniors to preserve their strength, balance, and overall health. However, several typical barriers can make it difficult for them to maintain a consistent fitness regimen.

1. Managing Pain While Exercise

Many seniors struggle to exercise because of pain. It can result from a variety of causes, including arthritis, past injuries, or ordinary bodily wear and tear. Knowing the difference between discomfort and pain is critical. While modest discomfort is typical during physical activity, acute or prolonged pain may indicate a need for caution.

One of the most efficient strategies to deal with discomfort is to listen to your body. If a workout causes pain, it is critical to adjust it or seek an alternative. If a regular squat causes pain, try a sitting leg lift or a wall squat. This permits you to use your muscles without stressing them.

A consultation with a healthcare physician or physical therapist might provide personalized insights into pain management. They can offer workouts or changes that are tailored to your personal needs, allowing you to continue exercising safely.

Low-impact exercises, like resistance band workouts or mild yoga, might be especially beneficial for seniors who are in discomfort. These activities help to alleviate joint tension while also increasing strength and flexibility. For example, resistance bands can give a regulated and adjustable technique to build muscles without the impact of weights.

Heat or cold therapy can be used before and after exercise to assist relieve pain. Heat helps relax stiff muscles, and ice packs can alleviate inflammation after exercise. Incorporating these therapies into your daily routine can help you stay active despite discomfort.

2. Overcoming Fatigue

Fatigue can sometimes be a substantial impediment to regular exercise for seniors. It can be caused by a variety of circumstances, such as drug side effects, medical disorders, or the natural aging process. Identifying the underlying causes of weariness is the first step toward finding answers.

One effective strategy to overcome fatigue is to choose the optimal time of day to exercise. Many people have variable energy levels throughout the day, so determining when you feel the most alert and energetic can greatly improve your workout experience. For some, this may be in the morning after a good night's sleep, while others may find that mid-afternoon is more convenient.

When weariness is an issue, it is critical to start small. Shorter, more doable workouts can be more successful than longer, stressful sessions. Aim for 10 to 15 minutes of activity per session, gradually increasing the duration as your energy level improves. Gentle exercises, such as stretching or modest resistance band workouts, can assist increase endurance without causing severe exhaustion.

Rest days are equally vital as workout days. Adequate recuperation time allows your body to regenerate, lowering the danger of burnout. On rest days, use mild activities like leisurely walking or gentle yoga to keep your body moving without overexertion.

Proper nutrition and hydration are crucial for maintaining energy levels. Eating balanced meals with a variety of carbohydrates, proteins, and healthy fats helps supply the energy required for exercise. Furthermore, staying hydrated is critical for sustaining energy and avoiding weariness, particularly during workouts.

3. Dealing with Lack of Time

Many seniors find it difficult to exercise regularly due to a lack of time. Workouts can easily fall to the bottom of the priority list when life gets hectic. One of the first steps toward overcoming this problem is to rethink your daily schedule. Identify periods when you can engage in physical activity, such as during a commercial break while waiting for a meal to prepare, or while on the phone.

Mini workouts, or little bursts of movement throughout the day, can be an excellent method to keep active without devoting a significant amount of time. For example, doing a few resistance band exercises while watching TV or doing easy stretches while on the phone will help you incorporate activity into your daily routine. Aim for at least three 5-10 minute exercise sessions spread throughout the day.

Combining social activities and exercise can also be an effective method to keep active while spending time with friends and family. Consider starting a walking club, attending a light yoga class, or participating in community fitness activities. These activities encourage social connection while also helping you achieve your fitness goals.

Setting reasonable and attainable workout goals might help you maintain focus and motivation. Instead of aiming for an hour of exercise every day, set a target of three brief sessions per week. Celebrate each accomplishment, and progressively expand your goals as you become more accustomed to your regimen.

Making a weekly fitness routine will help you prioritize workouts in a hectic lifestyle. Treat these sessions as essential appointments, and strive to adhere to the scheduled timings. Consistency is essential in developing a habit, and having a regular schedule might make it easier to stick to.

While pain, exhaustion, and a lack of time can be difficulties for seniors who want to continue an active lifestyle, they are not insurmountable. You can overcome these obstacles by listening to your body, consulting with professionals, determining the best time to exercise, and including little workouts into your daily routine. Remember that the idea is to remain active and interested in your fitness quest, even if that means changing your strategy. Prioritizing your health and well-being will allow you to reap the numerous benefits of regular exercise.

Real-Life Testimonies And Success Stories To Inspire

Real-life testimonials and success stories are effective motivators in the fitness and wellness industry. They provide hope, inspiration, and practical proof that good change is achievable, particularly for seniors seeking to enhance their health and well-being with resistance band activities. We'll look at some amazing stories from people over the age of 70 who have changed their lives thanks to resistance band training.

---

1. Mildred's Journey

Mildred, a 72-year-old retiree, had always lived a pretty inactive existence. After a slight fracture from a fall, she grew more hesitant to engage in physical exercise for fear of future injury. Mildred's daughter, concerned about her mother's health, introduced her to resistance band exercises.

Mildred was initially hesitant, questioning her ability to perform even the most basic actions. However, with her daughter's encouragement, she began attending weekly classes intended exclusively for senior citizens. The instructor stressed safety and perfect form, allowing Mildred to acquire confidence gradually.

After a few weeks, Mildred noticed noticeable changes. She was not only stronger, but her balance had improved, and she felt more enthusiastic all day. Her initial panic dissipated, and she felt a new sense of empowerment. Mildred now engages in group workouts twice a week and discusses her experience with others at her local community center, urging them to try resistance bands.

2. Frank's Transformation

Frank, 76, had always enjoyed hiking and spending time outside. However, following knee surgery, he found it increasingly difficult to participate in things he formerly enjoyed. Frank, frustrated and feeling limited, was eager to restore his strength and mobility.

He discovered resistance bands through an online exercise forum for seniors. Initially skeptical, Frank decided to give it a shot, purchasing a set of bands and following along with online lessons. The soft, low-impact aspect of the workouts made them more accessible, and he liked how readily he could modify the resistance to fit his strength level.

Frank's condition improved dramatically in just a few months. His strength had returned, allowing him to cross difficult terrain and climb hills once more. He even finished a 5-mile hike with pals, which he hadn't done in over a year. Frank credits resistance band training with giving him his life back, and he now urges his classmates to be active and try new types of exercise.

3. Mrs. Evelyn's Success

Mrs. Evelyn, 71, had recently lost her husband and was dealing with emotions of loneliness and melancholy. To overcome this, her doctor suggested she take a local fitness class. Mrs. Evelyn, skeptical but ready to try, discovered a senior-focused workout program that included resistance bands.

Initially, she felt out of place among the other participants, but the warm atmosphere put her at ease. The group immediately formed a support system, with members encouraging one another during each session. Evelyn gradually found herself not only becoming physically stronger but also developing friendships that lifted her spirits.

The joy she experienced in exercising with others rekindled her passion for life. Evelyn now attends lessons three times a week and has even taken on leadership responsibilities in her group, such as planning social events and recruiting new members. Her tale exemplifies resistance band training's all-around benefits, including physical health, emotional well-being, and social connection.

4. George's Revival

George, a 74-year-old former athlete, had serious health issues, including high blood pressure and weight gain. After years of inactivity, he was overwhelmed by the notion of returning to a fitness regimen. A friend introduced him to resistance bands, emphasizing their versatility and convenience of usage.

George reluctantly began incorporating exercise bands into his routine. He began with modest exercises for his upper body and gradually graduated to lower body and core training. To his astonishment, he discovered that he could complete several workouts without hurting his joints, allowing him to gain strength while remaining comfortable.

Over time, George observed a considerable drop in his blood pressure and an improvement in his energy levels. He lost 20 pounds, which gave him the motivation to continue his fitness adventure. Today, George promotes resistance training among his friends and family, demonstrating that it is never too late to accept change and enhance one's health.

5. Linda's New Chapter

Linda struggled with her identity after retiring at the age of 68. With her children growing and living independently, she sought other sources of fulfillment. Resistance band exercises became her solution. Linda was intrigued by their versatility and enrolled in a local fitness class for seniors.

Linda was initially driven by a desire to stay active, but she soon discovered a greater purpose. The sessions not only helped her physical condition but also revived her desire to serve others. Inspired by her experience, she chose to become a certified fitness instructor for seniors, specializing in resistance band training.

Linda currently teaches seminars in her neighborhood, sharing her knowledge and pushing participants to strive beyond their limits. Her story demonstrates how resistance band workouts can change people's lives, instilling not only physical strength but also a revitalized feeling of purpose and community involvement.

The success stories of Mildred, Frank, Evelyn, George, and Linda demonstrate the dramatic influence of resistance band training on seniors over the age of 70. These testimonials are a reminder that age should not be an impediment to physical activity or personal development.

Each narrative emphasizes the accessibility and versatility of resistance bands, demonstrating that everyone can embark on a fitness journey, regardless of their starting point. Real-life experiences can encourage others to take the first step toward a healthy lifestyle, instilling hope and motivation in people of all ages.

As more seniors discover the benefits of resistance band exercises, they not only improve their physical strength, but also foster resilience, camaraderie, and a thriving community dedicated to health and wellness. These stories inspire all seniors to embrace exercise, reminding them that it is never too late to begin the journey to a better, healthier, and more fulfilling life.

CHAPTER 10: COOL DOWN AND RECOVERY

The Importance Of Cooling Down After Workouts

Cooling down after a workout is an important part of any training routine, yet it is often disregarded or rushed. Many people are quick to finish their workout and move on to the next chore, but taking the time to cool down can dramatically improve recovery and help prevent injury.

Cooling down is the slow transition from high-intensity exertion to a resting state. This procedure entails slowing down your activities and engaging in gentle motions or stretches. A cool-down time usually lasts 5 to 15 minutes, depending on the intensity of the workout and the individual's fitness level.

High-intensity workouts like jogging, strength training, and aerobics cause considerable increases in heart rate and breathing rates. Blood flow is directed to the muscles being used, while waste products such as lactic acid accumulate. A proper cool-down allows the body to gradually return to its resting condition, facilitating effective recovery and minimizing potential issues.

Benefits of Cooling Down

1. *Gradual Heart Rate Reduction:* One of the key advantages of cooling down is a steady decline in heart rate. Sudden cessation of strenuous physical exercise can result in blood pooling in the extremities, causing dizziness or fainting. Allowing your heart rate to gradually decline benefits cardiovascular health and ensures proper blood flow throughout your body.

2. *Prevention of muscle soreness and stiffness:* Cooling down helps to avoid muscle pain and stiffness, which can develop after strenuous activities. Performing modest stretching and mobility exercises during the cool-down period helps to preserve flexibility and range of motion. This practice increases blood flow to the muscles, which aids in the clearance of metabolic waste products and lowers the risk of delayed onset muscular soreness (DOMS).

3. *Enhanced recovery:* The cool-down phase improves recovery by increasing the flow of oxygen and nutrients to the muscles. As your heart rate progressively drops, blood flow returns to normal, allowing your muscles to mend and recover more efficiently. This technique is especially crucial for individuals who exercise regularly because it helps to maintain performance levels and avoid overtraining.

4. *Reducing injury risk:* By gently relaxing your body out of high-intensity activities, you lower your risk of injury. A quick stop can cause strains or sprains, particularly in the muscles and joints. Cooling down helps to retain muscle elasticity and joint flexibility, making you less prone to injury in future sessions.

5. *Psychological benefits:* Cooling down allows you to reflect on your workout and mentally prepare for the remainder of the day. This phase can help you develop mindfulness and improve your overall exercise experience. Taking a few seconds to recognize your efforts might help you develop a positive relationship with exercise and maintain consistency in your habits.

Physiological Changes While Cooling Down

During a workout, your body goes through various physiological changes. To provide oxygen to muscles, the heart pumps quicker and breathing becomes more laborious. As you calm down, these processes eventually return to their resting state.

1. *Heart Rate Recovery:* According to research, faster heart rate recovery after exercise is linked to improved cardiovascular health. Cooling down permits your heart to gradually return to its usual rhythm, which can improve heart function over time.

2. *Muscle Temperature Regulation:* Muscle temperature rises during exercise, which promotes suppleness and efficiency. However, extreme heat can cause weariness and reduced performance. Cooling down allows your muscles to restore to their optimal temperature, lowering your chances of overheating and developing heat-related disorders.

3. *Hormonal Balance:* Exercise causes the release of several hormones, including adrenaline and cortisol. These hormones aid in energy mobilization during exercises, but they might cause tension if levels remain elevated after strenuous activity. A cool-down regulates hormone levels, facilitating relaxation and healing.

Effective Cool-Down Strategies

To optimize the benefits of cooling down, try combining the following tactics into your routine:

1. *Gradual transition:* Begin by lowering the intensity of your activity. If you've been running, turn to walking for a few minutes. If you've been lifting weights, reduce the weight and do the exercises with less resistance.

2. *Stretching:* Use mild stretching to target the primary muscle groups worked during your workout. Hold each stretch for 15–30 seconds without bouncing. Stretching improves

flexibility and range of motion, which are important for general fitness.

3. *Hydration:* Drinking water or a low-calorie sports drink will help you replenish the fluids lost throughout your workout. Proper hydration promotes healing and prevents cramps.

4. *Deep breathing:* Include deep breathing exercises in your cool-down. This technique not only helps with relaxation but also regulates heart rate and promotes mindfulness.

5. *Foam rolling:* Using a foam roller can assist in relieving muscle tension and discomfort. Spend a few minutes rolling out tight regions, concentrating on any discomfort or tension you may be experiencing.

Cooling down is an important part of any workout program, especially for seniors or those who perform high-intensity activity. By taking the time to properly cool down, you can improve recovery, lower your risk of injury, and promote overall physical and mental health. Incorporating slow movements, stretching, and drinking into your cool-down regimen can provide long-term advantages, ensuring that you maintain your fitness levels while enjoying the process of being active. Remember that a few minutes spent cooling down can make a big impact on how your body feels and works in the days ahead.

Breathing Techniques For Post-Workout Recovery

Breathing techniques are essential for post-workout recovery, as they promote relaxation, increase oxygen flow to muscles, and improve overall well-being. *Here are a few simple breathing methods that seniors can integrate into their cool-down practice:*

1. Diaphragmatic Breathing

Diaphragmatic breathing, also known as abdominal breathing, is the process of taking deep breaths with the diaphragm. This approach improves relaxation while increasing lung capacity.

How to Practice:

1. Sit or lie down comfortably, one hand on your chest, the other on your abdomen.
2. Inhale deeply through your nose, letting your abdomen rise while your chest remains motionless.
3. Exhale slowly through your lips, feeling your stomach drop.
4. Repeat for 5-10 breaths, concentrating on the movement of your abdomen.

This approach relaxes the nervous system, lowers anxiety, and increases oxygen flow to the body.

2. 4-7-8 Breathing

Dr. Andrew Weil created this approach to promote relaxation and reduce tension and anxiety.

How to Practice:

1. Sit or lie down comfortably, keeping your back straight.
2. Inhale gently through your nose for a count of four.
3. Hold your breath for the count of seven.
4. Exhale entirely through your mouth, generating a whooshing sound for the count of eight.
5. Repeat the pattern for four breaths.

4-7-8 breathing reduces heart rate, and blood pressure, and promotes a sensation of relaxation.

3. Box Breathing

Box breathing, also known as square breathing, consists of four equal parts: inhalation, holding, expiration, and holding again. This approach helps to regulate breathing and alleviate anxiety.

How to Practice:

1. Sit comfortably, feet flat on the floor.
2. Inhale through your nose for a count of four.
3. Hold your breath for 4 counts.

4. Exhale slowly through your mouth for a count of four.
5. Hold your breath again for a count of four.
6. Repeat this pattern for 5 to 10 breaths.

This practice improves concentration, lowers tension, and gives you more control over your breathing.

4. Pursed Lip Breathing.

Pursed lip breathing reduces your breathing rate and improves ventilation, making it especially beneficial after exercise.

How to Practice:

1. Inhale slowly through your nose for two counts.
2. Purse your lips as if you were going to whistle.
3. Exhale slowly and gently through pursed lips for a count of four.
4. Continue for 5–10 breaths.

This approach promotes oxygen exchange, lowers shortness of breath, and relaxes the body.

5. Progressive Muscular Relaxation (PMR)

PMR combines breathing and muscular relaxation techniques to relieve stress throughout the body.

How to Practice:

1. Find a comfortable sitting or laying position.
2. Take a big breath in and contract the muscles in your feet for 5 seconds.
3. Exhale to relieve the tension in your feet.
4. Tense and relax each muscle group in your body (legs, abdomen, arms, shoulders, and face).
5. Finish with a few deep breaths, focusing on your body's calm state.

PMR promotes relaxation, relieves muscle tension, and increases body awareness.

6. Mindful breathing

Mindful breathing raises awareness of each breath, promoting a sense of serenity and presence.

How to Practice:

1. Sit comfortably, eyes closed, or slowly gazing at a location in front of you.

2. Focus your attention on your breath, watching its natural rhythm without attempting to change it.
3. If your mind wanders, softly return your focus to your breathing.
4. Continue for 5–10 minutes.

Mindful breathing improves brain clarity, reduces stress, and promotes feelings of well-being.

Incorporating these breathing techniques into post-workout recovery regimens can be quite beneficial for seniors over 70. Individuals who focus on breath control can improve relaxation, increase oxygen flow to muscles, and build a stronger connection with their bodies. Diaphragmatic breathing, box breathing, and mindful breathing all contribute to a holistic approach to healing, supporting both physical and emotional wellness.

Managing Soreness And Preventing Overexertion In Seniors

As we become older, maintaining an active lifestyle becomes increasingly crucial for our general health and well-being. Resistance band workouts are a low-impact technique to improve strength, balance, and flexibility, particularly in seniors. It is critical to control discomfort and avoid overexertion during workouts in order to maintain safety and long-term physical activity. This tutorial explains how to manage pain and avoid overexertion, guaranteeing a pleasurable training experience.

Understanding soreness

Soreness, particularly delayed onset muscle soreness (DOMS), is frequent when beginning a new workout routine or increasing intensity. DOMS often develops 24 to 48 hours after exercise and might be characterized by muscle stiffness, soreness, or a dull aching. Soreness in seniors can be more severe due to age-related changes in muscle mass and healing capacity.

It is critical to distinguish between normal soreness and discomfort that may suggest an injury. Normal soreness often feels like muscle fatigue and can be relieved with light movement, stretching, and adequate rest. In contrast, sharp, sudden, or persistent pain may indicate an injury and should be evaluated by a healthcare professional.

The following are effective strategies for managing soreness:

1. ***Start slowly and progress gradually:*** One of the most effective ways to manage soreness is to begin any new exercise routine gradually. For seniors, this means starting with beginner-level exercises and gradually increasing the intensity, duration, and resistance. For example, when starting with resistance bands, start with lighter bands and fewer repetitions, then gradually increase as your body adapts.

2. ***Incorporate rest days:*** Rest days are necessary for recovery. Schedule at least one or two rest days per week, depending on your level of activity. On rest days, try low-impact activities like walking or gentle stretching to improve circulation without straining your muscles.

3. ***Stay hydrated:*** Hydration is critical for muscle recovery. Drinking plenty of water before, during, and after a workout helps to flush toxins and promotes optimal muscle function. Aim to drink at least 8 glasses of water daily, or more if exercising vigorously.

4. ***Utilize active recovery techniques:*** Active recovery techniques involve gentle movements that promote blood

flow without stressing the muscles. Incorporating activities such as walking, light yoga, or stretching can help alleviate soreness and aid recovery. Resistance band stretches targeting the sore areas can also be beneficial.

5. ***Warm up and cool down properly:*** Warming up before workouts prepares the body for exercise by increasing blood flow and flexibility, reducing the likelihood of soreness. Spend 5-10 minutes engaging in light aerobic activities (e.g., walking in place) followed by dynamic stretches. After exercising, cool down with static stretches targeting the muscles used during the workout. This practice helps to relax the muscles and reduce soreness.

6. ***Use ice and heat therapy:*** If soreness persists, consider using ice or heat therapy. Ice packs can reduce inflammation and numb soreness if applied for 15-20 minutes after intense workouts. Heat therapy, such as warm compresses or heating pads, can help relax tight muscles and promote blood flow to sore areas after the initial soreness has subsided.

7. ***Listen to your body:*** Listening to your body is paramount. If you feel persistent soreness, fatigue, or discomfort, it may be time to scale back your workouts. Pay attention to your body's signals, and don't push through pain. If necessary, consult a healthcare professional or a physical therapist for personalized guidance.

Preventing Overexertion

Overexertion occurs when physical activity exceeds an individual's capabilities, leading to fatigue, injury, or burnout. For seniors, overexertion can result from inadequate conditioning, improper exercise techniques, or unrealistic fitness goals.

Recognizing the signs of overexertion is crucial for preventing injury. Symptoms may include:
  - *Extreme fatigue*
  - *Shortness of breath*
  - *Dizziness or lightheadedness*
  - *Increased heart rate or palpitations*
  - *Muscle pain that worsens rather than improves with movement*

If you experience any of these symptoms, it's important to stop exercising immediately and allow your body to recover.

Below are effective Strategies for Preventing Overexertion:

1. ***Set Realistic Goals:*** Setting realistic fitness goals is key to preventing overexertion. Consider factors such as age, fitness level, and any pre-existing health conditions when establishing your goals. Aiming for gradual improvements over time will keep you motivated and reduce the risk of injury.

2. *Incorporate Variety into Your Routine:* Including a variety of exercises in your routine helps to prevent overuse injuries and boredom. Combine resistance band workouts with other low-impact activities like swimming, cycling, or walking. This diversity will keep your workouts enjoyable while ensuring you use different muscle groups.

3. *Follow a Structured Program:* Consider following a structured exercise program designed specifically for seniors. Many community centers, fitness studios, and online platforms offer senior-friendly workouts that provide guided routines tailored to individual fitness levels. These programs often incorporate warm-ups, cool-downs, and rest days to prevent overexertion.

4. *Prioritize Form Over Quantity:* When performing resistance band exercises, prioritize proper form over the number of repetitions or intensity. Incorrect forms can lead to injuries and increase the risk of overexertion. If unsure about your technique, consider working with a qualified fitness instructor who specializes in senior fitness.

5. *Track Your Progress:* Keeping a workout journal can help track your progress and identify patterns that may lead to overexertion. Note the exercises performed, the resistance used, and how you felt during and after the workout. This

practice will help you make informed decisions about adjusting your routine as needed.

6. ***Engage in Regular Check-Ins with Healthcare Providers:*** Regular check-ins with healthcare providers or physical therapists can ensure you're on track with your fitness goals and address any concerns about soreness or overexertion. They can provide tailored advice based on your unique health needs.

Managing soreness and preventing overexertion is essential for seniors engaging in resistance band exercises. By adopting strategies such as starting slowly, listening to your body, incorporating proper warm-up and cool-down routines, and setting realistic goals, seniors can enjoy the benefits of exercise without the risk of injury. Remember, consistency is key, and a gradual approach will yield the best long-term results for strength, balance, and overall health.

CONCLUSION

As we near the end of our tour through the world of resistance bands, it's important to consider the transforming effect of adopting these adaptable instruments into your exercise regimen, especially for seniors over 70. Throughout this book, we have looked at the several benefits of resistance band training and provided you with practical exercises to improve strength, balance, and mobility. By now, you should understand how resistance bands can help you live a better, more active lifestyle.

We began by addressing the core benefits of resistance band exercise, which is specifically designed for seniors. These bands provide low-impact workouts that successfully increase strength without the jarring impact associated with traditional weightlifting. This is especially important for older folks who may be coping with joint concerns or simply want to stay in good physical condition as they age. Resistance bands' adaptability enables a variety of exercises that target different muscle groups, increasing overall fitness.

You've learned how to choose the proper resistance bands for your specific needs and ability levels. These tools can be adjusted from light to heavy resistance as your strength increases. This adaptability allows you to begin with the fundamentals and proceed to more complex exercises at your speed, ensuring that your workouts are both demanding and realistic.

We also stressed the need to warm up and cool down. Engaging in these techniques not only prepares your body for exercise but also helps with recuperation and injury prevention. Warm-up procedures in your workouts are an investment in your long-term health, ensuring that your muscles and joints are prepared for the task at hand.

You've learned workouts developed for different fitness levels: beginners, intermediates, and advanced practitioners. Each session was designed to build on the preceding one, allowing you to acquire a solid foundation in resistance band training. We looked at seated exercises for people with limited mobility and more dynamic movements for those who want to push themselves farther. This framework symbolizes our dedication to diversity, acknowledging that fitness is not one-size-fits-all.

Customizing your resistance band routine is essential for sustaining motivation and interest. You are more likely to stick with your fitness journey if you create a training plan that is tailored to your objectives, tastes, and lifestyle. Remember, consistency is essential. It is not about how much time you spend working out; it is about incorporating exercise into your daily routine.

In addition to specific routines, remaining motivated is essential. You've learned how to overcome basic barriers like weariness, time limits, and minor injuries. By recognizing these obstacles and devising solutions to overcome them, you empower yourself to keep going forward. Real-life testimonials and success stories from other seniors have shown that age is no barrier to fitness. Their stories serve as strong reminders that it is never too late to begin exercising or adopt a healthy lifestyle.

As you continue to train with resistance bands, keep in mind the long-term benefits of these exercises. Improved strength, balance, and mobility lead to a higher quality of life, allowing you to carry out daily tasks with greater ease and confidence. Improved muscle tone and joint health can lower the chance of falls, which are a significant worry among older persons. The more active you are, the easier it will be to keep your freedom and continue to enjoy your favorite hobbies.

Physical activity provides significant mental health advantages. Regular exercise can improve your mood, reduce anxiety, and enhance cognitive performance. As you add resistance band training into your daily routine, you may notice that you feel more energized and optimistic about your health and well-being.

To stay on track, make clear, attainable training goals. Whether it's completing a particular amount of sessions per week, learning a new activity, or simply boosting your strength and endurance, having defined goals will help you grow. Remember to celebrate your accomplishments, no matter how minor. Each step you take toward better fitness is a win worth celebrating.

As you develop your program, remember to listen to your body. Pay attention to how you feel during and after your workout. Adjust the intensity and type of exercise as needed, always prioritizing safety and comfort. Your fitness journey should be motivating, not daunting.

Finally, realize that you are not alone in this path. Engaging with a group of like-minded people can provide both motivation and accountability. Consider attending local fitness courses for seniors, participating in online forums, or simply working out with a friend or family member. Sharing your experiences with others will help you stay motivated and enjoy your workouts more.

Resistance band training provides seniors with a simple, effective technique to improve their physical health and quality of life. With the skills and knowledge presented in this book, you may embark on a rewarding fitness journey. Accept the changes that come with increasing strength, balance, and mobility, and let them inspire you to live a lively, active life.

The fitness journey is a lifelong endeavor that can begin at any time. By introducing resistance bands into your routine, you are taking a significant step toward maintaining your health, independence, and happiness in life. So, break out your resistance bands, get moving, and reap the many benefits of an active lifestyle.

Your future self will appreciate you.

Made in United States
Orlando, FL
08 July 2025

62763566R00085